# The Cancer Warrior Handbook

MICHELLE PAMMENTER YOUNG

Illustrations

SARA MORTIMER

Copyright 2013 © Michelle Pammenter Young

All rights reserved.
Except as permitted under the U.S. Copyright Act of 1976, no part of this publication may be reproduced, distributed, or transmitted in any form or by any means, or stored in a database or retrieval system without the prior written permission of the publisher.

www.pammenteryoung.com
info@pammenteryoung.com

ISBN-10: 1492134651
ISBN-13: 978-1492134657

The author Michelle Pammenter Young herby exclude all liability to the extent or permitted by law for any errors or omissions in this book and for any loss, damage or expense (whether direct or indirect) suffered by a third party relying on any information contained in this book,

Credits:
The author wishes to personally thank the following people for permission to print their stories. Kathleen S Dukes, Patricia Stoop, Janine Dahmen, Patricia Turner, Ashley Blair Doyle and Rebecca Hunwardsen

CreateSpace Independent Publishing Platform
Printed in the United States of America

Cover and Internal Artwork © Sara Mortimer
Author photograph © Gadbois Photography

The information provided in this book is designed to provide helpful information on the subjects discussed. This book is not meant to be used, nor should it be used, to diagnose or treat any medical condition. For diagnosis or treatment of any medical problem, consult your own physician. The publisher and author are not responsible for any specific health or allergy needs that may require medical supervision and are not liable for any damages or negative consequences from any treatment, action, application or preparation, to any person reading or following the information in this book. References are provided for informational purposes only and do not constitute endorsement of any websites or other sources. Readers should be aware that the websites listed in this book might change.

The information contained in this book is not a substitute for qualified medical advice. The opinions expressed are based on my personal experiences with cancer and some of the treatments given to heal cancer. Please consult your personal physician for personalized medical advice. This book is designed to share experience, bring a little humour and shed a little light on what life is like with cancer.

# CONTRIBUTORS

The following people have kindly contributed their stories for this book. The hope is that you will get some inspiration from their individual journeys and perhaps find some new ways to get through yours.

Kathleen S. Dukes: Kathleen Dukes is a grown up Valley Girl from California born and raised. She is an accomplished hair designer who hated to give up her design work to become a Warrior. But a Warrior she became. You will mostly find her in the middle of her friends and family whose numbers are many.

Patricia Stoop: Patricia is a ferocious cancer cougar who lives in Whistler, BC with her ski bum superman husband, two children and two dogs. She is passionate about her work as a home care Occupational Therapist and loves walking in the mountains and anything to do with crafts. She has been a cancer warrior since 2011 and is currently living with metastatic breast cancer while fiercely advocating for medication coverage for herself and others with Stage 4 cancer.

Janine Dahmen: Janine is a G.I.S Technician (cartography), self-confessed techie and avid sports fan. Whenever possible, she combines her passion for photography with her love of travel. Born and raised in South Africa, Janine now makes her home in Vancouver, Canada.

Patricia Turner: Patti is a primary school teacher and a cancer survivor. She grew up in Nelson, BC and now resides in Dawson Creek, BC. Her two grown children, her husband of 33 years, and her black lab named Molly, helped her to get through the hardest battle of her life.

Rebecca Hunwardsen: Born and raised in Merced, CA, Becca is a 27 year old who loves shopping, swimming, going to the beach, the gym and hanging out with friends and family. She has a degree in rehabilitation counseling and works in the field of counseling services.

Ashley Blair Doyle: Ashley is a graphic designer, foodie and creative Jill-of-all-trades. She was diagnosed with breast cancer at 28 and began blogging about her kicking cancer crusades in January of 2012. She lives on British Columbia's beautiful Sunshine Coast with her awesome husband and two crazy felines.

## DEDICATION

This book is dedicated to all the men and women out there who are currently fighting cancer, to those loved ones who have fought the battle and lost, to those who have fought the battle and won and to those who may still have to face the beast.

It is my hope that one day cancer becomes a disease of the past. Until that time, we need to be strong and fight.

# CONTENTS

|   | Introduction | i |
|---|---|---|
|   | "Today is Not the Day" a poem by Laurie Dewar | v |
| 1 | Becca's Battle | Pg.#2 |
| 2 | Finding the Blessings in Ovarian Cancer | Pg. #7 |
| 3 | Living with Recurrence | Pg. #10 |
| 4 | The Fight for Life | Pg. #17 |
| 5 | The Worst Kind of Thyroid Cancer | Pg. #24 |
| 6 | Kicking Cancer - one day at a Time | Pg. #29 |
| 7 | The ABC's | Pg. #39 |
| 8 | Life Lessons | Pg. #93 |
| 9 | Beyond Cancer | Pg. #97 |
| 10 | Resources | Pg. #100 |
| 11 | A note to the reader | Pg. #106 |
| 12 | Excerpt from "The Year I Died" | Pg. #107 |

# INTRODUCTION

Dear Reader,

I am glad this book has found it's way into your hands. The unfortunate thing is this probably means you are struggling with cancer or you are a caregiver of someone facing cancer. This little book will hopefully answer some of your questions and be a little helping hand as you go through the process of dealing with cancer.

As a fellow cancer person and currently a new survivor I know only too well what you must be feeling as you begin on this long journey. You will go through the usual stages of anger, denial and disbelief followed by rage, shock and frustration. There will be so much questioning going on. Not just the "why me's" that go on in your head, but also questions from other people, even your loved ones, who mean well, but some of their questions may be upsetting for you. To answer the question as to why this happened to you. They may say things like, "well didn't you smoke way back then?" or "do you think what you ate or drank had anything to do with it?" It will be frustrating for you and in most cases we can never pinpoint a "why", nevertheless we humans will still try to find an answer that makes sense. You see for your friends to come to the understanding that it just "happened" is scary for them. What it means to them is that if it happened to you without cause, then it can happen to them.

So while all this may be difficult for you, in most cases everyone means well, they are just scared, like you are. Your journey may be long and challenging, so make sure to surround yourself with the supportive friends, the ones who love you and who don't care why this happened, who only care that you will be okay and who will bend over backwards to help you over the next few months.

Each cancer diagnosis comes with a unique set of stages that you have to go through in order to recover. For the lucky ones, this may only be a small lumpectomy or excise surgery to remove the tumor. For most of us however the journey will involve, chemotherapy, surgery and radiation. It may involve long-term oral chemotherapy or hormones after the initial treatment, and may even involve bone marrow transplants or other invasive procedures.

Regardless of your treatment regime, a cancer diagnosis is a terrible blow. It is like here you are slowly riding your relaxing cruiser bike down a lovely trail, enjoying the deep woodsy odours around you, immersed in the beauty and the sounds of the birds when suddenly you run face first head on into an invisible glass wall. Suddenly everything changes; nothing will ever be the same. You no longer hear the birds or smell the peaty ground all you can think is what the hell? Why Me? Life stops dead in its tracks.

You have to find your way around this invisible wall. It will be a long hard journey and you cannot do it alone. Your doctors and the amazing nurses will help you on the medical side, your friends and family will support you at home and on the practical side, but you need to work on the emotional, spiritual side. I promise you there will be days where you don't want to live, don't want to continue going through the hell it may take to recover. I also promise you that if you keep putting one foot in front of the other, keep getting up out of bed, keep fighting for your life and your sanity, you will make it to the other side. It is well worth it once you get here. I am not the same person I was before I got sick, and you won't be either, but the person you will become is so much brighter than the one who came before. You will see life differently and your priorities will change. The person who emerges will be beautiful and you must realize there is no going back, only forward to a better fuller life.

I hope this book will be a good guide to get you there. It is divided into a few sections. The first section consists of a compilation of short stories from other Cancer Warriors. The second section is the ABC's of cancer treatment and symptoms that result from the treatment. The comments are meant to inform with humour and honesty. This is information you will not get from your doctor. This is from those who have walked the road before you. The third and final section is a listing of places where you can go to meet others still walking this journey. This is for you to reach out if and when you feel you need to.

I have done my best to include the most pertinent information here regarding side effects and things you may possibly go through, but obviously, since I have not experienced it all, I cannot possibly include everything, so I would love to hear from you if you can add any helpful tips to future editions of this book

This book, like a life after cancer is a work in progress. It is put together with love and help from other warriors, so please enjoy it and please recommend it to others who may need a little uplifting during their journey.

All the best.

Hugs,
Michelle

MICHELLE PAMMENTER YOUNG

THE CANCER WARRIOR HANDBOOK

## Today Is Not That Day

Tomorrow might be harder than I thought.
Hopefully learning all the lessons that were taught.
Letting go of body to encompass more of Soul
Embracing Soul Transcendence was always the goal.
It's not always easy to say goodbye to all I have been.
I have done it many times or so it would seem.
I hope I can make this transition with all the love I have found
And leave the world behind where temptations abound .
The Heavenly Realms are calling, singing a far off song.
Promising a home where I have always belonged.

But that is not today for today I am here
In a land of opportunity present and clear.
Life is a precious gift not one moment will I miss.
I have more to learn of love so the heavenly song I must resist.
The pursuit of life, love and true happiness continues without falter
To experience all the wonder and the joy this world has to offer.
God has a plan for me to which I must surrender.
I have to keep going one foot in front of the other.
My heart needs to open more to follow His command.
I place my love, my life, my heart, my body in His hand.
When it's all been said and done and all the lessons learned
I'll follow the Heavenly Song to home
Where my Soul is at last returned.

But today is not that day!

Laurie Dewar
Dx Sept 30 2011 with IBC

# WARRIOR STORIES

# BECCA'S BATTLE

On March 8th, 2013 my life turned upside down. At 26 years of age I was diagnosed with Breast Cancer. To be more specific, I had Triple Negative, Stage 2, Grade 3 Invasive ductal carcinoma. A few months prior to my diagnosis, I had felt a lump. I followed up on this, as my mother had breast cancer a few years prior, and was told after an ultrasound that I simply had a cyst and it would likely go away on its own.

However, after a few months, it didn't, instead, it got larger and harder. I followed up, and was again told it was a cyst, however after trying to get it "aspirated," found out the lump was a solid mass. I was told it was very unlikely cancer, due to my age, and likely fibroid breast tissue. However, that was not that case.

On March 8th, the day after my biopsy, I received the call while I was at work. The radiologist first asked how I was feeling, then told me, and I will never forget this moment, his voice and the fear I felt, as he stated, "well, you do have a cancer there." I got hot, couldn't breath, and went into organized mode, staying calm, asking questions as to what came next and drove to my parents home, where once I was off the phone, and came in hysterically crying, waking my mom up, she knew what it was and she broke down. I will never forget her face, her voice and seeing the fear she felt for me.

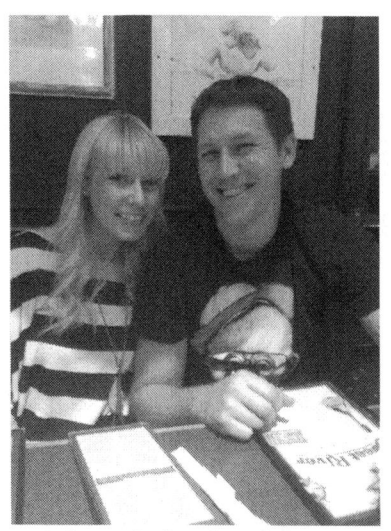

Rebecca before her diagnosis

We called my immediate family that day, I asked my boyfriend to come home early from work and he knew. I informed many of my close friends. It was very hard to tell people at first.

The next few weeks, things moved fast, as I had an aggressive cancer. Within two weeks, I had met my oncologist, got a heart scan, a lymph node biopsy, got my chemo port put in, had a PET scan and started chemotherapy. For me, knowing I had to have chemo was very scary, as I already had a hair condition that caused my hair to grow slowly and thin, so I was devastated knowing I would lose my hair.

Preparing for chemo, what helped keep me sane, was keeping very organized, preparing for what to expect and doing everything I could to prevent the side effects. My boyfriend, roommate and I started a strict schedule with keeping our house very clean, stocked up on good lotions, hand sanitizer, wigs, hats, cancer cook books, etc.

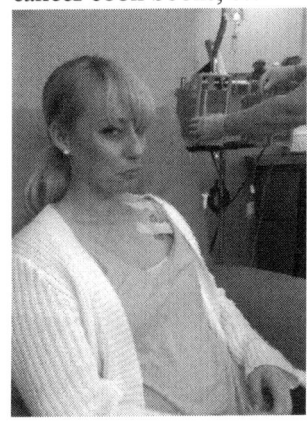

During chemo I learned to chew on ice and soak my nails (both hands and feet) in ice water during infusion to prevent nail changes. I was on what is called the ACT treatment, which is Adriamycin, Cytoxin and Taxotere. I had 6 rounds of this, having 21 days between each treatment.

Becca at her first chemo

Chemo really was not what I expected, and overall was not as bad as it used to be in the old days, or those horror stories I would hear. As my doctor said, having young age on my side really helped me. I experienced side effects, but very few. Of course I lost my hair, got hot flashes, gained weight (from the steroids), but I never got sick, nauseated or anything that prevented me from doing things I enjoyed (and with icing my nails, I didn't lose them! Great trick). Throughout my almost 4 months of treatment, I continued to work, except for around treatment time, I went on trips on my good weeks, when my white blood cell count was going back up. I had a ton of support, from my family, boyfriend and friends. We did a ton of fundraising to help pay for my treatments (because, having cancer is expensive!). I felt pretty good at least two thirds of the time.

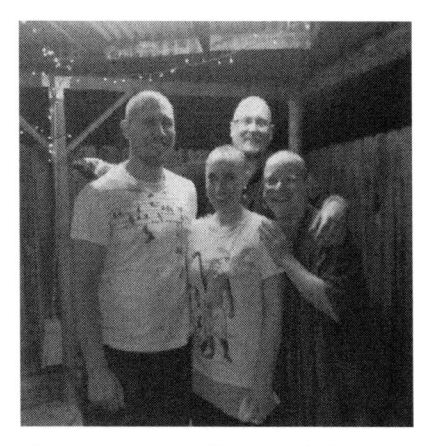

The day Becca had her head shaved.

I had my last chemo treatment on July 8th, 2013. I think coming to the end of this phase was both relieving, yet scary. Knowing the drugs that had been actively fighting my cancer, and had been decreasing my tumor size over time (as I couldn't even feel it now), wouldn't be in my body anymore, was scary. Chemo kind of became my security blanket. I learned to enjoy my time after chemo, feel like a normal (now) 27 year old, and enjoyed summer while I could, as I had another step in my treatment coming up.

I made the choice to have a double mastectomy with reconstruction. As I currently write this, I have not yet had my surgery. But, I am very nervous and scared and also can't wait to get it over with and have the joy of really saying I am cancer free.

In asking questions and getting information, I have come to terms with my choice and feel it is the best for me, not only to living a full life, but to ensuring I am living a life not looking over my shoulder, wondering, "oh hey, is that you, cancer?"

My advice to anyone going through this, is don't be scared

to still live your life. You are not your cancer; you are still so many other things. I made sure to not isolate myself or make excuses; I still made sure to enjoy the time I felt well doing things I loved. I learned to cope through humor, making jokes about being bald and about my hot flashes. I learned to love wearing wigs, the quick and easy time it took to get ready and do my "hair." I found a lot of comfort and support through online forums, cancer groups and connecting with others my age who were going through it, both to connect emotionally but as well as to ask questions and know what to expect for my future.

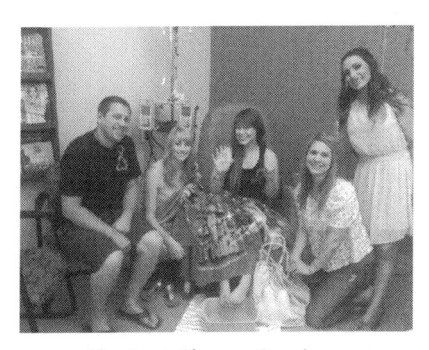

*The Last Chemo Session*

Most people seemed surprised at how well I coped, saying I was inspiring, or handling it "so well." Well, yes I did handle it overall pretty darn well (if I do say so myself, all things considered), but I still had bad BAD days. The days where I would sob off and on, worry about everything, think about dying, ask "why me?" over and over, but it does get better. It does pass and you do learn to cope.

I suppose being a pretty optimistic, rational thinker normally also helped (as well as being a counselor in my profession, I learned to practice what I preached). However I allowed myself to feel crappy too, and that's okay. One thing I will say is DO NOT GOOGLE. Google is not your friend, and it will tell you that your body is riddled with cancer. Don't do it. Trust me. You will get unsolicited advice from others who are not healthcare professionals. They mean well, they do, but it will get annoying. Learn to listen, thank them, and ask your doctor or research their thoughts if you're interested.

I still have a long road ahead of me. Though I wouldn't wish cancer on my worst enemy, having cancer does make you appreciate life, the important things and teaches you to not sweat the small things. Through this journey, I feel I have matured, became wiser, stronger and experienced more than most. I have made what I hope is lifelong connections and strengthened my relationship with God in the process.

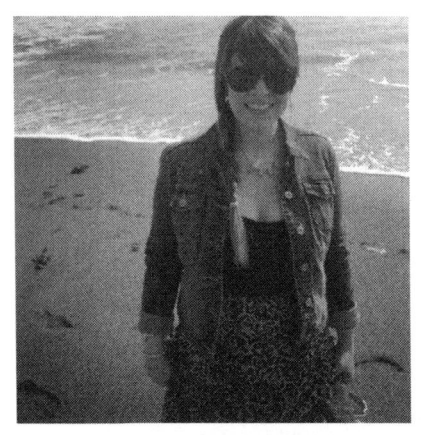

Rebecca Hunwardsen, Cancer fighter and soon to be survivor, 27 years old.

Rebecca two weeks after her last chemo

www.beccasbattle.wordpress.com

# FINDING THE BLESSINGS IN OVARIAN CANCER

## KATHY'S STORY

My name is Kathy Dukes and I am an Ovarian Cancer survivor. Before my diagnosis I was a social hard working hairdresser with full appointment books, wife, mother, grandmother, photographer, gardener and loyal friend. I have scleroderma so autoimmune issues seem to follow me around. I have always been a positive person that made friends easily but I lacked a confidence that upon diagnosis asserted itself and I became a true Warrior.

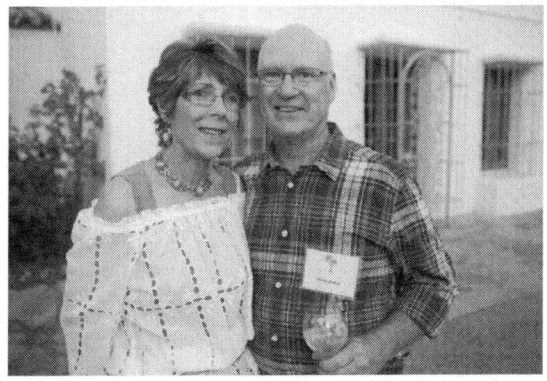

*Kathy and her husband prior to her diagnosis*

I became a different person something like when Clark Kent ripped his shirt off and became Superman able to leap tall buildings. I was on a mission. I was not going to die from this disease.

I was diagnosed on June 12, 2012 with a hysterectomy for a cyst on my ovary that had started to grow. My GYN called in a GYN oncologist surgeon just in case and I knew. My diagnosis was ovarian cancer stage 1C that means both ovaries were involved and my left ovary had ruptured. When is anyone's guess?

If I've learned anything on my journey I have learned that faced with a major life crisis you step up to the plate. Your back becomes straighter and your priorities change. I chose not to surrender instead I wanted to be an inspiration.

Being a Hairdresser I also wanted to teach women how to be stylish when in chemo with no hair. I found that attitude is everything. When you looked better you felt better. I noticed people started to gravitate towards me. I reached out I held hands. I became the Wal-Mart greeter of my chemo room.

I had six chemo treatments that took its toll on my blood so I had to have 38 blood and platelet transfusions. The chemo caused MDS. Oh boy a new auto immune issue. My spleen became extremely enlarged because it was now trying to make up blood production for my bone marrow that was barely working.

My support system was so great that it made me stronger. Proven statistics show that good support systems for cancer patients give them better survival rates. I educated myself so that I could teach other young women what the symptoms of ovarian cancer are and to become aware and proactive with their own bodies.

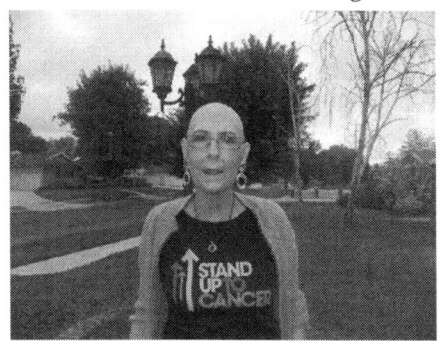

Kathy during chemo. Still Rockin it!

If I had not been proactive we would not have found my cancer at stage 1, which in ovarian cancer is very important. It is called the silent killer because it is not usually found till stage 3 or 4. It does have whispering symptoms. I have become a vocal advocate for the women's cancers. I have made friends around the world. I have joined cancer forum support groups and made friends with other cancer survivors.

Reach out! There is so much support out there. Cancer is Cancer you have now become a member of a special group of Warriors that are fighting also.

Tell your story.

My Doctor has been my Guru and lifesaver. My Nurses are now good friends, my cancer center is like home to me and they are my new family. I will be a patient the rest of my life as MDS is a permanent blood disorder.

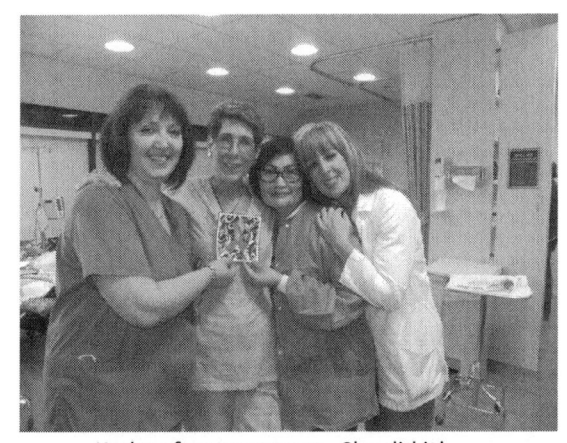

This may sound crazy but Cancer has been a real blessing in my life. I am now Cancer Free and am a strong, confident, happy Ovarian Cancer Warrior that will try and make TEAL the new Pink.

Kathy after treatment. She did it!

I'm alive today to make a difference and I'm well on my way.

You can follow me on Pinterest under Kathleen Dukes it gives many style tips and where to go for hats, scarves, wigs, different ideas to make chemo and radiation easier for your skin and nails.

Fist up you new WARRIORS~

You can do this.

I send you Love and Strength on your new journey. Turn your negatives into positives and find your blessings too.

Fist up, Kathy!

# LIVING WITH RECURRENCE

# PATRICIA'S STORY

Believe!

I am a forty something year old mom and home care Occupational Therapist in a small city of BC, Canada.

My story starts like many breast cancer stories do. I found a couple of smallish lumps in my breast one day in the spring of 2011 at the age of forty. I went to the doctor and what followed was a whirlwind of scans and appointments.

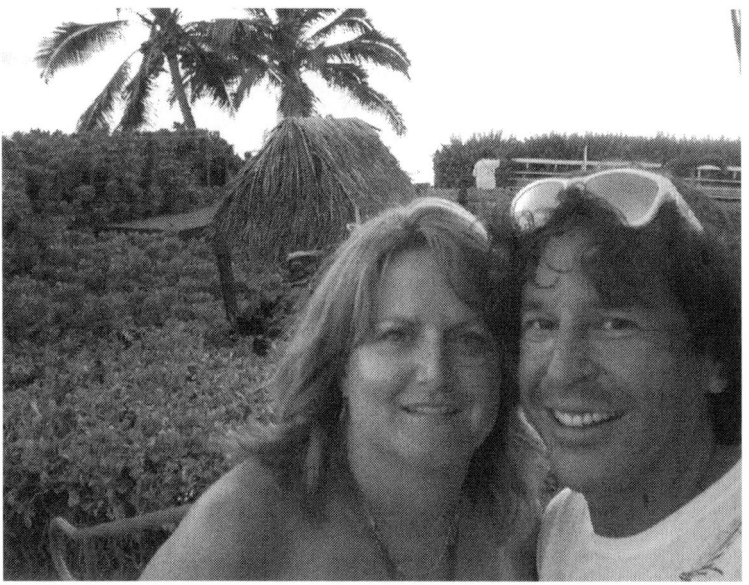

Patricia with her husband in 2010 before her diagnosis.

The results finally came in and I was diagnosed with a particularly aggressive locally advanced Her-2 cancer with lots of lymph involved. The tumours had grown from two lima beans to at least four masses 8 cm or more over six weeks. I underwent chemotherapy for six months, had a left mastectomy with lymph dissection, a right mastectomy, radiation and then continued Herceptin chemo for over a year.

I learned to meditate and started to move towards a more vegetarian diet, I participated in work conditioning and a gradual return to work. I had my share of complications and rough patches but I always believed I would overcome cancer. I had a number of follow up scans and was told I was cancer free in August of 2012.

I went for a six-month review in April 2013. I was singing, "I'm on Top of the World." I was working full time again and loving it. I had just been to Hawaii to celebrate the end of treatment with my family. I was exercising again. I really thought I was finished with cancer forever. I thought I was going to be able to post a picture of me holding "In remission" on my Facebook page.

Then the world dropped out from under my feet when my oncologist told me my blood work showed cancer. I would need a full body scan and I would likely need to start chemo ASAP. Within a few days all the scans were done and I received the call at work that I had extensive liver metastases and liver lymph involvement. Surgery was not an option. He would write the orders for chemo and wanted me to start on a brand new drug called Perjeta. It held the most promise in available treatments for metastatic HER2 cancer. The issue was the funding but an assistant from the drug company would help me. I was able to start chemo that same afternoon and onwards I went to conquer cancer again.

Now hearing I had cancer the first time was pretty awful and scary. Well hearing I had it again and it was metastatic was a hundred times worse. I was frozen with fear and often broke into tears. I was furious with God. I needed sedatives to survive the evenings with the kids. I screamed then cried myself to sleep for a couple of weeks. I wondered if the pain would ever subside. I didn't fear death for myself but for my children, my husband, my family, friends, colleagues and clients. It was so unfair that my children had to go through mommy being very sick all over again. It is SO damn unfair.

One evening shortly afterwards we were watching a very sad but beautiful movie about triumph against the odds. My husband told me that I had to fight cancer and BELIEVE in my treatment. That was the turning point for me. I did believe that medicine could be filled with miracles, that a higher power was working for us and that I could become a cancer warrior once again.

I was the second person in Canada to receive Perjeta funded by my benefits. I made a sign on my way down to treatment that said, "believe" and took photos with it and posted it all over social media. "Believe" became my slogan. All around the world we had people praying or sending us positive vibes.

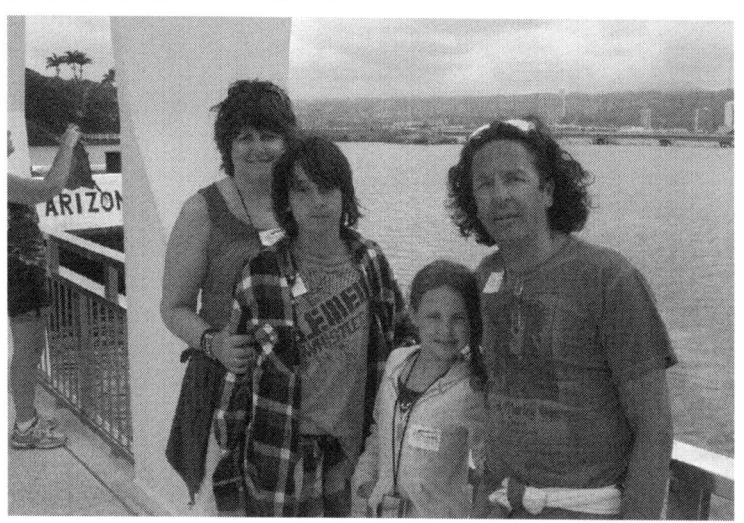

Patricia with her family before her recurrence.

Then, once again, someone pulled the world from under me. My contract changed and my extended benefits would no longer cover my medication. At a cost of $3500 a dose every three weeks for the rest of my life I knew continuing my treatment would not be possible. Again I was in despair. I called around with the help from my funding assistant at Big Pharma. All this negotiating became a full time job.

In my research I came across the process of getting new oncology drugs funded in Canada. They are first approved for use then reviewed at both a federal and provincial level to determine if the province will fund them. This process can take 2-3 years. Seriously. If you have metastatic cancer you may not live long enough to benefit. I decided to enter the world of advocacy. I was not going to take that lying down. I would approach the governments and tell them to hurry up the process so more people can live.

In the meantime I continued to negotiate my coverage one dose at a time. Between my benefits, my husband's benefits and the drug company I have negotiated about a year's worth now. Hopefully Perjeta will be closer to provincial funding by then. I also have friends involved in some great fundraising initiatives. I am blown away with love and gratitude.

For now there are many unknowns in my future. I anticipate living with metastatic cancer as a chronic disease that will require some form of treatment for the rest of my life. I want to raise my children, return to work in some capacity and leave a legacy with respect to advocacy. There are no guarantees - I could just as easily be killed in a car accident as killed by my cancer returning with a vengeance. So I must truly learn to live one moment at a time and try to be mindful in each moment. A pretty monumental task I must admit.

A few keys to success for me:

- Support network: I have the most amazing network of family, colleagues, friends and neighbours that want to help. It took some getting used to asking but now I realize how my support network is key to my success.
- Believing treatment is going to work - it doesn't matter what drug I am on, what alternative or complementary treatment I try. The act of believing itself has very powerful healing properties in my opinion.

- Leaning to meditate. Cancer is the roller coaster from hell. Meditation is a great tool for riding it with some grace. Moments of true peace are few and far between but are worth the effort.
- Self-Compassion: I can get wound up in the whole guilt, blame, and fear cycle. I can be positive and kick ass. Every emotion is fair game. Sometimes I go for counseling for help.
- Self-Advocacy - I have always been direct, honest and inquiring with my treatment team. I don't take anything lying down. I research my options and I negotiate.
- Be "nice" to my team. I can get frustrated and angry but I try to always be thankful and diplomatic. MY team will do anything for me because we have a trusting and respectful relationship.
- Informed decision-making: The Internet is a scary place. I suggest staying away from it until you are stronger and know a bit about your disease. There is a lot of untrue or questionable information out there about cancer. Lemon juice or soursop is not going to cure my metastatic cancer. Anyone can write whatever he or she wants about cancer without research or editing. I personally detest the conspiracy theories - they are not healing. I research, look at all sides, cross-reference. I try to have an open mind with people who propose alternative methods as superior to traditional. I have my own belief system about what will work but I openly adopt aspects of healthy living that I feel are right for me and will help me heal.

I am a work in progress; I will continue my battle with my head held high and love in my heart.

I BELIEVE!

I am a survivor!

## Tips from Patricia:

What's worse than being told you have cancer?

It's being told on your two-year remission apt that you seem to have cancer again but they don't know where it is. So you play the scan-n-test-n-wait game again but it's way worse and way scarier.

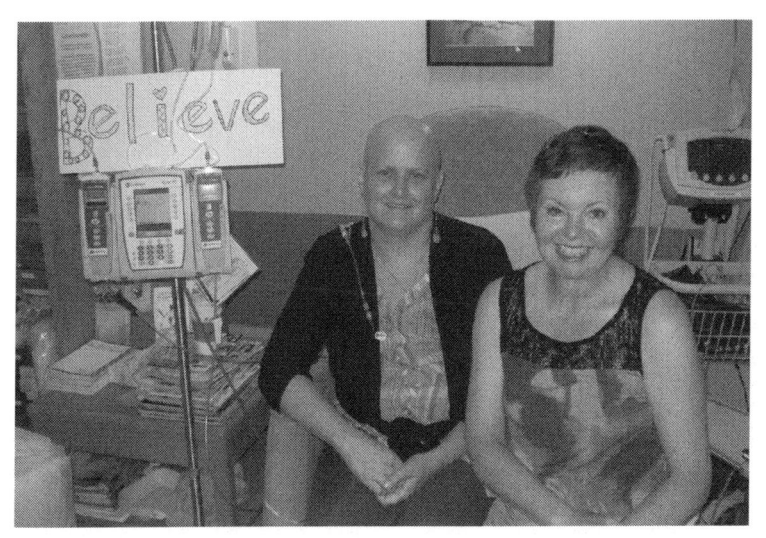

Patricia during her current treatment.

Strategies to survive the waiting game:

(This applies to new any diagnoses or recurrences)

Start checking out other women's boobs - look for the ones you want your plastic surgeon to create. My friends let me touch theirs.

Buy the perfect, cute, sexy bra and hang it up - that's your goal.

Have sex - take your time and lead in with a super long body massage or sexy book ("Fifty Shades" perhaps).

Hang out with girlfriends who can make you laugh and are convinced you don't have cancer - it was just a mistake in the labs.

Watch a funny movie - "Life at 40" had me almost peeing my pants.

Ativan - a new old best friend for those moments when you just can't pull it together

Zopiclone - little blue sleeping meds. You can't kick cancer's ass without sleep. Sleep is when you heal and so on.

Get a little support network together at work and try to work a bit. Filing, organizing and preparing for your potential coverage perhaps.

Lets the dogs sleep in your bed. To hell with dog hair

Try to follow your old routine. Get up on time to get the kids to school. Follow your bedtime routine.

Connect on social media with a group that can support you.

Buy a ukulele and learn to play somewhere over the rainbow. But pace yourself - it hurts fingertips if you play more than fifteen minutes at a time.

Run away and hide under the covers then just breathe - several times a day if needed.

# THE FIGHT FOR LIFE

# JANINE'S STORY

"Is there somebody here that you would like to have with you?" This, coupled with a visibly upset doctor, is not a question anyone wants to hear. Lucky for me, my boyfriend John was in the waiting area. As I waited for him to join me, I remember feeling my heart pounding so hard and fast that I thought it was going to jump out of my chest.

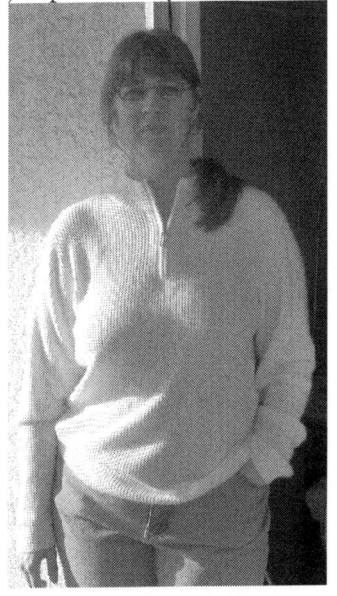

I had been to see my GP two weeks previously, the day before my birthday, as I was suffering from extreme fatigue and felt like I had some type of virus. I joked about my body objecting to turning another year older. I had blood work done and the results came back borderline for mono. My doctor didn't agree with that, so I had more blood tests and an ultrasound as I was experiencing slight abdominal discomfort. The ultrasound showed secondary cancer on the liver. Date of diagnosis: the 23rd of July 2008, two weeks after my thirty-ninth birthday.

**Janine before diagnosis.**

Blood tests, mammogram, bone scan and CT scan followed and it was discovered that the primary cancer was in the right breast, but had spread to the liver and bones. After a liver and breast biopsy it was determined to be HER2-positive.

I was informed that I would lose my hair, so to make things easier for me to manage; I had my hair cut before treatment started. My hair was quite long, down past my shoulders. I had it styled into a bob and donated the cut length for wigs.

First chemo was Thursday August 21st, 2008 with a second, different treatment the following day. I had an immediate reaction to the first treatment – started throwing up within a couple of minutes of them starting the IV. They halted the infusion, but continued with saline while they located a doctor to come and check me over. After some heavy-duty anti-nausea drugs, treatment was continued. Afterwards, I was taken to a ward and left to recover for a couple of hours before being released.

Treatment the next day was uneventful.

Exactly one week later, August the 28th, I started experiencing abdominal pain, beginning around lunchtime. It got progressively worse, so around six o'clock my mother called the Cancer Agency and left a message for the doctor on duty. The call was returned quite quickly and after questioning my mother, the doctor advised her to get an ambulance and have me taken to Emergency. Mom followed his instructions and I was taken to Lions Gate Hospital.

LGH was in the process of upgrading their Emergency section, so the place was a bit of a disaster zone. After about one hour, I was moved into the Emergency ward and from there taken for X-rays. I was finally given morphine and at around two in the morning I eventually fell asleep.

I vaguely remember a doctor visiting me the next morning and talking about putting me on a ventilator and in an induced coma. I was told that if I agreed, I might not ever come off life support. The reason for the induced coma being that the doctor felt that my chances of survival/recovery would be a little bit better than if I was just put in a bed upstairs in a ward. I was in a complete fog from the morphine, so requested that he contact my parents. He said they were on their way.

My parents arrived and I was already being prepped for the ICU. I remember telling my Mom that I was only thirty-nine years old and that we still had lots of stuff to do and places to see, and although I have cancer, this would not take over my life and I wouldn't allow it to take my life.

The doctor warned us that this could be the last time I ever spoke, or that my parents heard my voice.

Since I have almost no recollection of the following five weeks, my mother is my reference for all events.

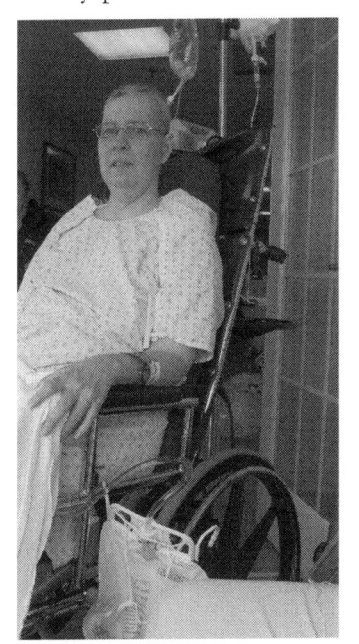

Janine Oct 2008

Whilst my parents were visiting me in the ICU on my first day in there (29th August), the nurse told them that a surgeon was requesting to speak to them. They were taken into a private room to see him and he said that he needed to do surgery on me. My mother inquired as to what type of surgery. He responded saying that I would have to have a total colostomy and he did not think I would make the surgery, as I was so ill and weak. My mother then asked what made him think I needed this surgery as nothing of the sort was mentioned while I was being prepped for ICU, and in particular the type of surgery he wanted to perform. She told him he wasn't going to do it, wasn't going to mutilate me and he was not to do the surgery. His reply was that I was dying and I probably wouldn't see the morning. My mother then responded that she is a believer in faith and if God wanted me, He would take me. The doctor asked my father whose response was also no to the surgery. My boyfriend John was also present. He said that even though he had no say, he agreed with my parents. My mother then requested that the doctor leave and said she never wanted to see him again!

Saturday morning, my parents again came to visit me. The doctor from Emergency, who had me admitted to ICU, said he believed that we'd had a visitor the previous night. He gave the thumbs-up sign and said my parents' decision was correct not to allow surgery on me. I was under the care of several doctors. My mother approached one of them and asked if he would speak to Dr. Klimo (Lions Gate Hospital's number one oncologist) on her behalf about taking me on as his patient. He did so and Dr. Klimo agreed, but said he could do nothing until I was out of ICU.

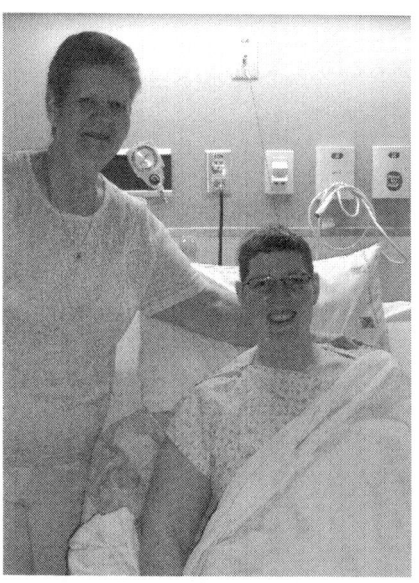

Janine & Evol (her mother and biggest supporter) July 2009.

I was heavily medicated with two drip stands and fourteen bags of drugs. I had a feeding tube, a central line, and PICC in my left arm. I was also suffering from extreme edema. The doctors were trying to determine exactly what was wrong. They knew I had a very severe infection, but were not able to pinpoint it.

My parents had been told to talk to me constantly, even if they repeated the same things. I could not respond, but I could possibly be aware of their presence. Since I was in an isolation ward in the ICU, John would sit with me and sing my favourite songs. I was brought out of the induced coma each day to be checked by the medical staff and then put back into the coma. Each night, at the end of their visit, my mother and John would have a big hug for luck. This practice continues to this day after my appointments with the oncologist (which is every 6 weeks).

A week into my stay in ICU, my hair started to fall out. My mother approached our hairdresser for assistance and she kindly came up to the hospital and cut my hair as best she could.

I was in the ICU for fourteen days. They took me off life support and removed the breathing tube around the 14th of September. I was then moved to the sixth floor to SCO (Surgical Close Observation unit). I was there for about three days before being moved down to the fourth floor, where I stayed for about ten days.

Around the 25th of September (almost a month after I had been admitted to the hospital), the doctor's finally discovered what they thought might be the problem – a perforated colon caused by a severe infection. The doctors said that the infection was caused by a drug they had given me on the 21st August, to which I was allergic. I was told that if I ever wanted to live a normal life and be able to eat again, I required surgery. I agreed to go ahead and the arrangements were made. By this time, I had lost about forty pounds in weight and was extremely weak. The surgeon warned my parents that I might not make it through the surgery. I said I was going through with it, and my parents and John supported me fully.

On Saturday, the 27th of September, my mother signed the documents giving permission for the surgery. I was taken to the OR at around one o'clock. My parents saw the surgeon at eight o'clock that night. He came from the OR with a big smile on his face and told them all had gone well and I was in recovery. The surgery was an ileostomy, and removal of eight inches of my colon. I was then taken back to SCO around midnight.

Since I couldn't move on my own, the nurses would have to turn me on my side and prop me up with pillows. The slow process of recovery began and I had physio every day. I couldn't sit unaided, or even get out of bed, so they would use a body sling and a bed lift to hoist me into a wheelchair.

Dr. Klimo arranged for me to have chemo and I was taken down to the Chemotherapy Clinic. Unfortunately, there was no bed lift there and I was not able to get out of the wheelchair without one. I was sent back to the ward and one of the

Chemotherapy Clinic nurses came up to SCO and administered the treatment.

I remained in SCO for about ten days, before being transferred to another regular ward on the sixth floor. Just before leaving SCO, my feeding tube was removed. I was being fed intravenously, one bag of food every 12 hours.

Physio continued as there was no bed lift in the regular ward, and I slowly progressed from wheelchair (where I initially could only sit for about ten minutes at a time) to walker, to walking stick, to doing the rounds using the IV pole for support. The intravenous food was removed and I was started on small amounts of liquid. My diet was gradually increased to include solid food, although I had a hard time feeding myself for the most part as I was so weak, I had very little control over holding a spoon or fork.

Along with learning to sit, eat and walk again, I was faced with the prospect of having to be trained on how to function with my ileostomy. The wound care nurses made sure it was healing and functioning correctly and the nurses had to empty it. As the time neared for me to go home, I was then taught how to empty it myself.

A week before I was due to leave the hospital, my parents were told they could take me home in a wheelchair, to begin the transition from hospital to home.

Finally that next week, the doctors agreed to discharge me and on Thursday, the 6th of November, I left the hospital. My ten-week stay in LGH was over.

After surgery, I had three drains attached to me. One was removed before I left the hospital, but I went home with two drains, a PICC line and an ostomy bag. Arrangements were made for me to receive home care nursing. This started on the 7th of November and continued until the beginning of December 2009.

Chemo started again and continued until September 2009.
After ten months, I had an ileostomy reversal, on the 15th of July 2009, almost one week after my fortieth birthday. Couldn't

have asked for a better gift!

The treatment was changed after my surgery and my hair grew back.

On the 2nd of December 2009, the PICC was removed from my arm and a Port-a-Cath was inserted into my chest. This was replaced on the 23rd of January 2013 as I continue to receive Herceptin every 3 weeks.

I look at this as my 'new normal'. I feel very fortunate to have recovered to the extent that I can now work part-time. Before my diagnosis I enjoyed travelling. I am happy to say that I am doing that again. This journey has been a life-changing event, and it definitely has a bearing on how I look at the world now. I am inclined to procrastinate less these days and am more willing to 'go and do'. I am also more aware of how precious time is; time spent with family and friends; time spent travelling and making new memories – all of these are very important. I have been, and remain, positive through it all as I believe this frame of mind enables me to accept where I am and to continue along this path, wherever it may lead.

As I approach 5 years since my diagnosis, I credit my parents and my boyfriend, John, for their incredible support for where I am today. My mother was and still is an incredibly strong advocate for me. My friends have also played a very important role. I am most grateful to Dr. Klimo, Dr. Smiljanic, and the wonderful medical staff at Lions Gate Hospital.

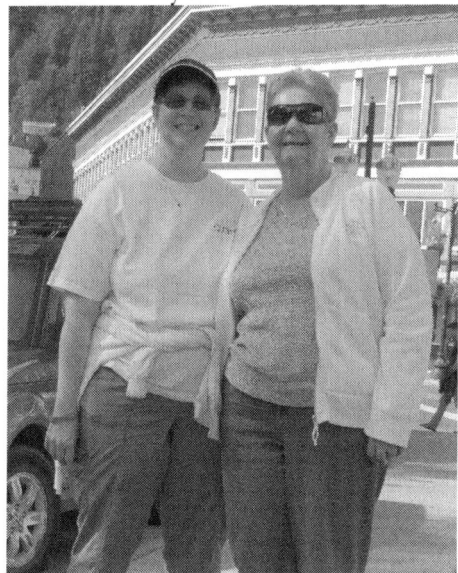

Janine & Evol July 2013.
5 years since diagnosis.

# THE WORST KIND OF THYROID CANCER

## PATTI'S STORY

My journey started with a lump in my neck. It wasn't a large lump. Most people couldn't even see it, but I could feel it. I saw my doctor early in June 2011 and he sent me for an ultrasound and a biopsy. The results of the biopsy showed hurthle cells. Hurthle cells need to be seen in order to make a diagnosis so I was scheduled to have the right side of my thyroid and the isthmus (the bridge between the two sides) removed on September 30, 2011. This surgery left me with a paralyzed vocal cord due to a damaged right laryngeal nerve, which meant I didn't have a voice. All I could do was whisper.

Two weeks later I was told that I had papillary cancer. The surgeon told me that if you have to get thyroid cancer that is the one you want. Hearing that information did not help. Cancer is cancer. He told me that the survival rate is good. But just to be sure, the thyroid tissue was then sent to Vancouver. I went on the Internet to learn all about the cancer. I proceeded to learn about all the different thyroid cancers. About ten days later, I went to my doctor to find out the final results. That was the day my life changed drastically. My doctor told me I now have anaplastic thyroid cancer. The really bad, very aggressive, thyroid cancer. From my research I knew anaplastic thyroid cancer was the worst. When you are diagnosed with this cancer you have 3-6 months to live. That is all. It is usually found too late. I was upset and in a state of shock. The report says I have three different kinds of cancer in my thyroid. The report went on to say "I have never seen a case like this and can find no useful literature on this entity." After I got a copy of this report I thought I didn't have a chance. I won't get to see my kids get married and I won't get to hold my grandchildren.

My doctor said I would need to get the rest of the thyroid removed. He also sent me for a CT Scan, which showed, thankfully, that the cancer had not spread to my chest. A surgeon at the University of Edmonton Hospital would remove the rest of my thyroid. Prior to the operation, I had a PET CT Scan, which also showed the cancer had not spread. That was very good news. During the second operation, the left side of the thyroid was removed and then the surgeon removed the damaged part of the right laryngeal nerve, but my voice didn't come back for many months. When it came back, my voice was raspy, but definitely better than the whisper.

Near the end of December, I had my first appointment at the Cross Cancer Institute in Edmonton. I would be having two treatments: radioactive iodine and 30 sessions of external based radiation.

At the beginning of January I went back to Cross. In the morning they had to make the mould for me to wear during the external beam radiation treatments. When they were making the mould on my body, I could not control the tears. Ever since the diagnosis I had prayed it was a mistake and that one day they would realize that. At that point, I realized I really had cancer. Later that day, I was admitted for the first treatment, radioactive iodine. This involved drinking the radioactive iodine and being in isolation in the hospital until my numbers got low enough to go home. The liquid was in a metal canister and I had to put on rubber gloves. I drank the liquid (which doesn't taste very good!) through a straw. I also had to sign a paper that told me I could end up with leukemia later in life due to this treatment. The nurse used an instrument to get a reading on my body and I was told it had to get down to a certain number before I got to leave the hospital the next day. I drank five and a half jugs of water and had four showers. The water and the showers helped to flush it out of my system. No one could come near me because of the radiation in my body. The next morning the nurse used the same instrument and it showed the level had dropped enough to let me go home. My husband arrived soon after. We then had a six-hour drive to get home. Luckily, we have a crew cab so I sat in the back seat on the passenger side. At that distance, I was actually still too close to the driver. At this time, I still had a paralyzed vocal cord so my husband brought a stick along to give to me to use to poke him in the shoulder if I needed to get his attention, as my voice was still just a whisper. Also, because my body was radioactive, I could not use a public washroom. We stopped along a few dirt roads when I had to go. I wonder if mutant plants are now growing in those places! We got home and had to keep our distance. I slept in our daughter's bedroom. If we were in the living room, I was in one corner of the living room and my husband was in the other. I used one bathroom and my husband used the other. Our son went to live at a friend's house for two weeks. Our dog Molly even went to live with a friend. A week later I had to return to Edmonton for a full body scan.

On February 13 we drove back to Edmonton. This time it is for the radiation. In Edmonton, there is a house called Compassion House where ladies can stay when they are going through cancer treatment. That is where I was lucky enough to stay for 6 weeks. I made some very good friends while staying at the house.

My first treatment was on Valentine's Day. My husband and I don't normally celebrate Valentine's Day, but this one was special. It was the day that I was starting the next part of my battle against cancer, the treatment that is going to allow me to be alive for many more Valentine's Days.

I was to have thirty sessions of radiation. My husband stayed with me for the first week. Two of my sisters came separately during the next two weeks. My husband returned for a few days. Then a very good friend from high school came to spend almost two weeks with me. She is a nurse and it was so helpful to have her there, both for the friendship and for the nursing knowledge.

My radiation basically went from the chin line to my shoulders. I had to lie on a table, then the technicians would put on the mould (it went from just under my nose to about 5 inches below the shoulders) and then it is strapped to the table. The table slides into the radiation machine. From what I understand, that is when they are getting everything lined up. Then I would be slid back out, the technician would push a few buttons and then I would be slid back in for the treatment. While I was getting the radiation, I would try to think happy thoughts. Thinking of my kids. Packing my suitcase for a cruise. Thinking of snowmobile trips with my family. Anything to get my mind off what was actually happening. The radiation, as it is happening, does not hurt at all. What hurts is when the tissue starts to be burnt. After about a week, food starts to taste like metal. After about two weeks, swallowing doesn't come very easily. After another week or two, swallowing is painful. The doctors prescribe medicine that helps a bit. About the end of week four, my doctor suggested I start to use morphine. At first, I said no because I was afraid to use it. My friend the nurse was with me at this time and she said that I should start to use morphine. I thought if she was there with me then nothing would go wrong the morphine did help a bit. But by this time I was really not eating much, nor was I drinking much water. Each morning I would eat three, very soft, boiled eggs. They would slide right down without too much effort. That was just about all I was eating, other than the odd spoonful of soft, mushy type food. I even tried baby food a couple times. I tried to drink Encore or Boost near the end of my treatments, but liquids hurt to swallow and everything tasted terrible. Of course, with all the medicines, along comes the constipation. Not pleasant, but I did get over that.

My daughter lives in Edmonton so we were able to spend a lot of time together. Many evenings she would come over and she would knit while I made jewelry or did my Zentangle drawings. I also planned ways to celebrate different stages of my radiation treatment. After ten treatments, my daughter and I went for a manicure. After 20 treatments, the reward was a pedicure. After the thirtieth treatment, and to mark the end of radiation, my husband, daughter and I went to see Blue Man Group. The next morning we came home. It was so nice to be home. I had missed my husband, my son and my dog.

I knew that the radiation side effects would continue to get worse until two weeks after the last treatment and that was true. The effects from radiation eventually did improve. My immune system was weak so I ended up getting shingles at the end of May.

I was supposed to do the radioactive iodine again at the end of June so I was taken off my thyroid medicine for the six weeks. I slowly began to get all the side effects associated with being off thyroid medicine. When I got to Edmonton I was pleasantly surprised to find out I did not have to have the treatment. My blood work was where it should be. My doctor called me a 'rare bird' because no one survives anaplastic cancer. He sent me for another PET CT Scan and it showed I was cancer free! Woohoo!

I have no salivary glands so always have a dry mouth. This has caused me to have issues with my mouth. Some of my taste buds are pretty well back to normal. I used to enjoy fruit, eating at least three pieces a day. Now, whenever I eat most fruit, it is like eating a ball of salt. I think it is the taste bud for sweets that is still not back to normal. From what I have read, it probably won't get any better. But I can live with this.

Now I go back to Edmonton every three months for my checkups. Each time I am there my doctor reinforces how lucky I am. In December 2012, he said I was 'making history' because the anaplastic cancer is 'universally fatal.' My appointment in June he said I was '1 in 100,000."

I now try to live each day like it is my last. I enjoy being with family and friends. I am thankful that I am the 'rare bird.' My advice to anyone diagnosed with cancer is to stay strong and positive. You can beat it!

If you are up to it, continue to exercise throughout your treatment. I like to run and I tried to run throughout my battle. Of course I couldn't run for a couple weeks after each surgery and when I was in Edmonton for radiation I chose to go for walks instead. The rest of the time I would run 4-6 km at least once a week.

Good luck and don't give up!

# KICKING CANCER - ONE DAY AT A TIME

# ASHLEY'S STORY

It was December 2011 when life completely changed. Living on British Columbia's Sunshine Coast in our sixth rental house in seven years of being together, Mike and I were in a pretty good space for the most part. We were just getting ready for the Christmas holidays, I was going on my fourth year working as a graphic designer at a community newspaper, Mike a carpenter for a local builder, both of us looking forward to an upcoming month long adventure to Indonesia in the new year.

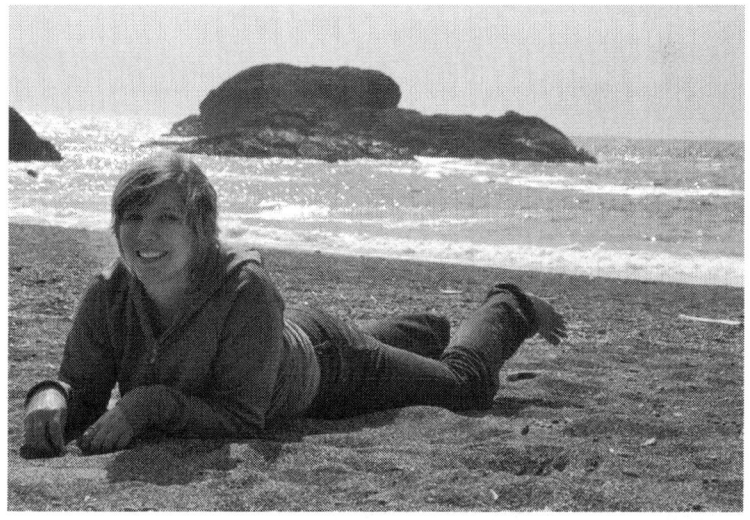

Ashley before her diagnosis.

Then the day following one of our staff Christmas parties I felt it. An alarming, undeniably there, hard lump in my left breast. I went to my GP first thing Monday where I was assured it was probably just a benign adenoma. These were common in young women and being twenty-eight years of age I didn't have any reason to worry about breast cancer. Since my GP was optimistic I felt reassured all would be fine. Because I wasn't concerned, I foolishly did not ask Mike to join me for my ultra sound that was scheduled a few weeks later. Big mistake.

Where one usually expects the ultra sound technician to do their thing and send you on your way without giving you any indication of their findings, I was met with a completely opposite encounter. Not only did the technician need to do my exam three times, the radiologist eventually came into the room and began to somberly question me about my family history of breast cancer. "We don't want to assume the worst Ashley... Have you been in a car accident or had some kind of injury to your chest recently?" "No," I said. "Has your mother or a sister had breast cancer?" "No," I said again. "Is there someone here with you in the waiting room?" "No," I said for the third time. "We need to do a mammogram." Shit.

After the infamous breast squishing and my first ever anxiety attack, I was told by the radiologist that a biopsy needed to be performed but that it would have to wait until the end of next week. Two days before Christmas. Lovely.

I think it goes without saying, that particular Christmas was the worst one of my life. The waiting was excruciating. The unknowns. The fears. The worst-case scenarios that played out in my mind and in Mike's. The late night cries. The visions of dying young. Along with the brutal task of keeping all of it a secret from my entire family so as not to have a dark cloud hanging over everyone's heads.

Then the call came on New Year's Eve. Not the one where they deliver your results over the phone but the one where the receptionist tells you that your GP would like to see you but you must wait the entire long weekend until the medical clinic is open again on Tuesday in order to find out that, yes, you have cancer. More waiting. More painful angst and time to think and worry and play out all the variations of the outcome in my mind.

The truth is, after that traumatizing ultrasound I knew it was going to be bad news. As much as we had hoped it wasn't going to be cancer, deep down my intuition was telling me I had a long hard road ahead.

Finally, the appointment day arrived. Mike came with me this time and we got the official diagnosis: Grade 3 Invasive Ductal Carcinoma. An aggressive kind of breast cancer. At 28 years of age. Happy flippin' 2012!

The next month was a whirlwind of appointments, phone calls and emails from concerned friends and family, chaperoned Google searches and more tearful late nights. I stopped working immediately and was thrown into medical world chaos feeling scared as hell but also ready and determined to gain control and know what we were up against.

So began what felt like endless days of cancer school. Surgeon. MRI. Fertility options. Bone scan. Medical oncologist. Radiation oncologist. Another biopsy. Cancerous lymph node results. Plastic surgeon. Abdominal ultra sound. Naturopaths. All kinds of cancer related books from friends, family and strangers even. Really good advice. Unwanted advice. Detoxes. Cleanses. The removal of emotional blocks. Forgiving past hurts. Reconstruction decisions. And then the choice to undergo a mastectomy.

Within a few weeks I had my surgery, which consisted of a complete mastectomy with immediate reconstruction (implant with Alloderm) and an axillary lymph node dissection (due to the known positive node). At the same time, I also opted for a breast reduction on my 'good' side so that I would be balanced with the newly created boob. So long big D's - hello not having to wear a bra! (Gotta look on the bright side, right?)

A week after surgery we learned that I did indeed have a grade 3, 100% estrogen positive, 2.8 cm tumour with 1 of 12 nodes involved staging me at 2b. Before I could catch my breath and come to terms with the loss of my breast, I was thrown into more decision-making. I began IVF to preserve embryos two weeks post surgery and then had to decide whether or not I would go through with the recommended 8 rounds of secondary-precaution-let's-make-sure-we-get-it-all chemotherapy. I struggled with this for weeks feeling sick to my stomach each time I thought of having to go through with it. I was not at peace with doing chemo. But I did it anyway. And it epically sucked. Obviously.

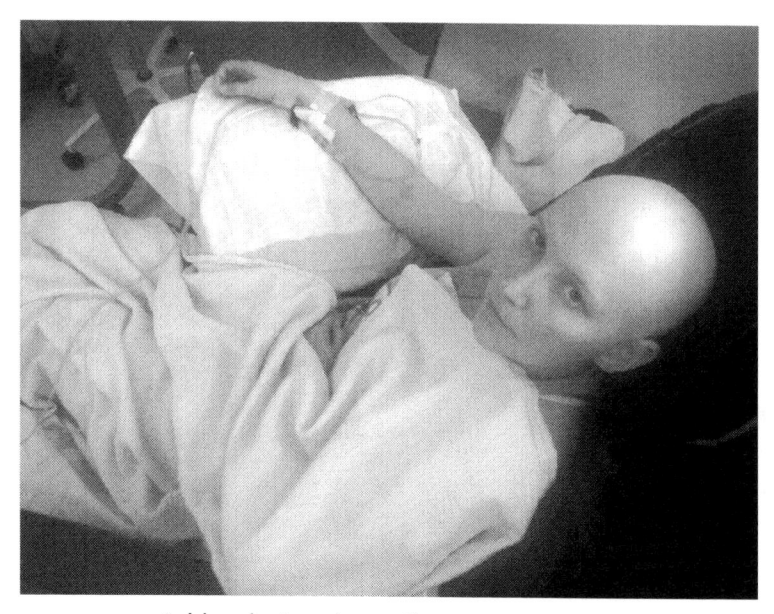

Ashley during chemotherapy treatment.

Due to the single lymph node being positive (with only .4mm of cancer! Seriously!) I had to entertain the idea of doing radiation therapy as well. Another not so fun decision to make. But I did that too. Eventually I made it out on the other side. Along with Benette, Harlow and Jenny - I am totally a geek and named my wigs :) Again, you have to make the best out of a shit-storm situation when you can!

Being a twenty-something year old dealing with breast cancer has been extremely difficult. I know cancer is awful at any age, but when you have your whole life ahead of you it is quite different because it is less expected. The reality of cancer and all that comes with it as a young person can be devastating. While most young ladies my age were having children, attending fun social parties or planning their next awesome trip to far off places... I was dealing with being bald, going through chemo-induced menopause, feeling like I was eighty years old, wondering if I would ever have children and worrying about whether or not I would even live to see my 30th birthday.

On top of the usual stresses that come with a cancer diagnosis, Mike was also let go from his job due to a work shortage during my six weeks of radiation. The financial strain has been rough. The relationship changes have been disappointing. The long-term side effects from treatment have been difficult. The Fatigue. Depression. Anxiety. Low libido. Isolation. Loneliness. Facing mortality. Uncertainty. Fear.

Then of course there is the point where you are told you are free to live your life. You've successfully completed all of your treatment (not including Tamoxifen for 5 years of course) and you are now told you can try and go back to somewhat of a normal life. Whatever that means.

Needless to say, the transition from cancer patient to cancer 'survivor' has been challenging for me (as it can be for many of us). But I try to take it day by day. Hour by hour even. Moment by moment if I have to. Things that have really helped me get through this uncomfortable limbo of reintrajectorization (aka: new normal) are: yoga, eating well, gardening, counseling, sharing and talking with other young adults coping with cancer (Young Adult Cancer Canada retreats are a must if you are 40 and under!), being the admin for a private cancer group on Facebook, exercising, writing my blog, doing creative projects and having someone solid in my life like Mike to help keep me sane.

Even though there have been a lot of really horrible things to overcome because of the big C, the fact is that we've also had a lot of good things happen too. Although these major milestones may have occurred anyway, I think cancer was somewhat of a catalyst to propel Mike and I into living life a tad more aggressively... We had been together for so long, it was about time we got engaged. So in between harvesting eggs/preserving 10 embryos and starting my first round of chemo Mike popped the question! With no wedding date in mind we made it through the grueling 4.5 months of dose dense AC/T treatment just wanting to get it out of the way and then eventually we would get to plan our big day. But doing heavily toxic drugs would not be complete without the purchase of our first home! Thanks to some major financial help from family, right smack dab in the middle of treatment Mike and I dove into real estate and bought the cutest rancher on a quarter acre. Some called us crazy for adding that to our list of things to accomplish during an already stressful time, but we did it and haven't looked back.

No, not all has been bad as a result of cancer. Throughout this roller coaster ride I have met so many incredible new friends, grown so much in my relationship with Mike and generally just learned a ton... how awesome my amazing guy is, how fragile our lives are, the importance of living in the moment, how hard it is for a parent to watch their kid go through hell, who our true friends are and that I really do have a lot more strength and courage in me than I had initially thought when all of this started. I would never go as far as to say that cancer was a gift. But without this life-altering diagnosis I would never have met a lot of the inspiring people I now call friends or learned as much as I have about life, other people and myself. For that I am grateful.

Now 19 months out from that traumatic January day where I thought that being told I had cancer was equivalent to being handed a death sentence, I am told I am cancer free. Although another mammogram exam is nearing for my one lone healthy breast, I am trying to live each day healthfully, peacefully, joyfully and with as little fear as possible... as hard as that is sometimes. I am also happy to say that my fake boob (aka foob) reconstruction has been completed by having a new nipple made out of my own skin and I have micro-pigmentation scheduled in a month's time to finish it off.

As for everything else that falls under the umbrella of my new normal after-cancer life... I am planning to return back to work soon, I am looking into studying holistic nutrition, we're chipping away at home projects, and Mike thankfully landed a new job... Also some happy news: Almost 9 years to the day, Mike and I tied the knot at the end of June. Oh and I recently celebrated my 30th birthday too! (Big smiles).

THE CANCER WARRIOR HANDBOOK

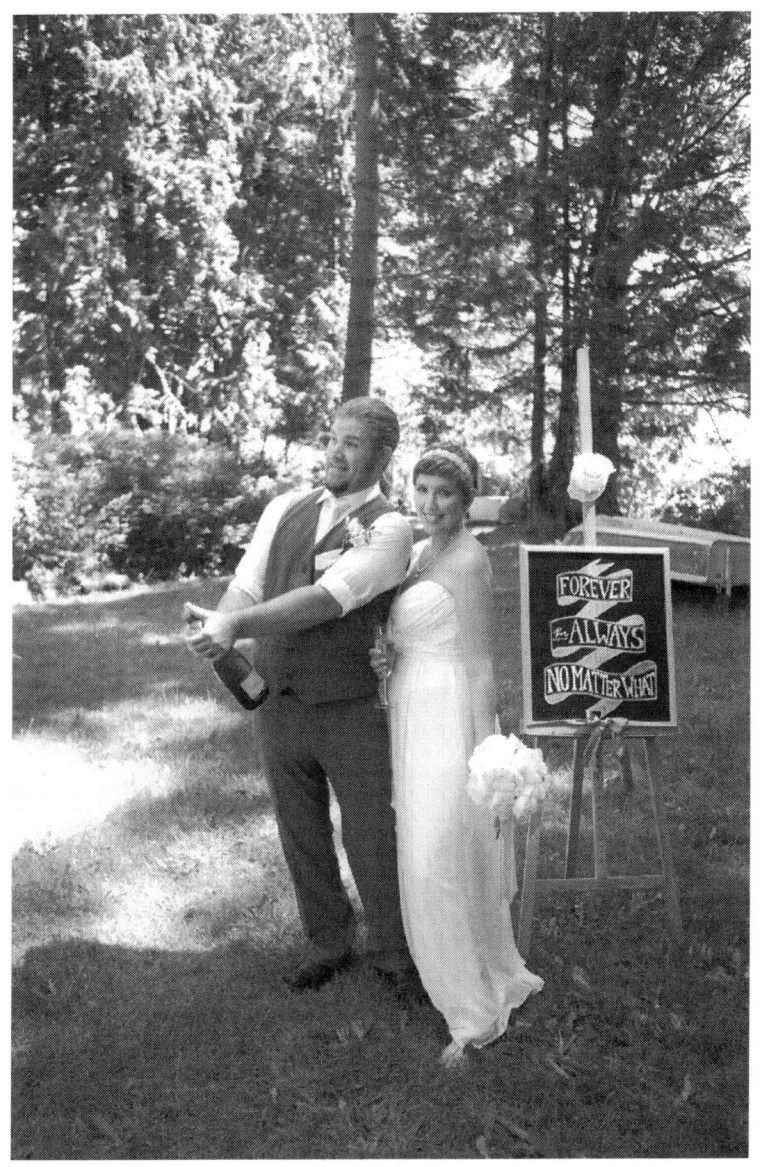

**The Big Day**

www.photophilcro.com - **Photography by Phil Crozier**

Life has definitely been turned around, thrown upside down

and tossed from side to side because of cancer. I've endured more than most people my age will ever have to and although I do find with time things get easier I am still trying to find my footing as I navigate through this uneven survivorship terrain. But each day I am thankful to be here, however tough it gets, I am determined to be happy and healthy, advocate, help others, share my story and continue to live life to the fullest.

You can find me on my blog page below
Ashley :-)

www.ashleykickingcancer.blogspot.com

# THE ABC'S

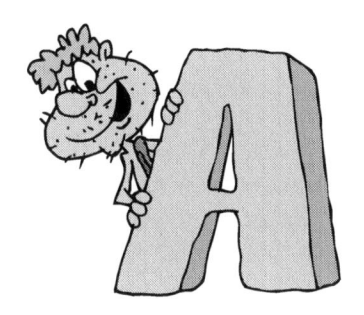

**Adriamycin:** (also known as Doxorubicin) is a drug used in chemotherapy. I call this Tiger's Blood (a dig at old Charlie Sheen). It is red in colour and typically administered via a huge syringe directly into your IV by a nurse. It is pushed in slowly because of the risk of an allergic reaction. This was in my opinion the worst of my chemo drugs. It caused severe nausea and made me feel sick from day two until about day six following chemotherapy. You will be given anti-nausea pre-meds prior to getting this drug, but make sure your doctor prescribes you some good anti-nausea meds for the days following. This drug can make your pee red and if you vomit it can be red too. Adriamycin will also make your hair fall out with a week or two of the first dose, something to look forward to.

Dear Caregiver: If your loved one has been given this drug, realize they will probably feel pretty sick for a few days. If they do vomit, make sure you wear gloves at all times to clean up. The drug can also give you metal mouth and mouth sores, I found fresh pineapple and Haagen Dazs Ice-Cream were good things to eat during this time.

**Appetite:** your appetite can go up and down like a seesaw during cancer treatment. Some people are hungrier and gain weight because of the steroids and inactivity. Some people completely lose their appetite and waste away. Try to eat regular, smaller meals and indulge in the odd treat if you want. Listen to what your body is asking for.

The cancer agency dieticians are mostly involved with serious weight loss and serious swallowing problems related to cancer and the treatments.

A good resource in some areas is for you is to call 811 for health information and ask to speak to a dietician about your cancer or treatment.

**Arts and Crafts:** Painting, sculpture, knitting, crochet, sewing, scrapbooking, woodwork and so on. If you can't work and don't want to be sucked into the Internet or TV vortex, find a crafty activity you love. Perhaps you can even work through some of the crazy emotions cancer brings. Look into Art Therapy if this resonates with you.

**Audiobooks:** these were a lifesaver for me. I am an avid reader and very shortly after my first chemo session I found I could no longer read. Now I'm not saying I lost my ability to read, rather, I lost the ability to focus for any period of time, and even getting through one paragraph in a book was challenging. I even tried to go from traditional books to eBooks and that didn't help. So, I decided to try audiobooks and I have been hooked ever since. My first foray into audiobooks was with Audible.com and although I still use them for most books, I have since found out that you can go online with your Public Library card and get free audiobooks through them. The selection is not as great as that at Audible, but then again, a free book is a pretty good thing.

Listening to audiobooks can do a couple of things for you. It can take your mind off the stresses you are going through, you can get lost in an amazing story and also it is a great tool to help you fall asleep. I usually set my book to automatically turn off after thirty minutes, typically I fall asleep a few minutes before it turns off and sleep like a baby. Often if I just tried to go to sleep without the book my mind would wander and I would never fall asleep.

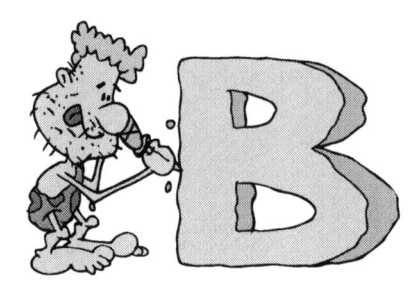

**Bone Pain:** this will be described to you as a dull aching pain that cannot be attributed to any specific bone. As someone who has experienced this, I would say that is baloney. Bone pain is a deep aching pain that you can feel in your bones, especially the larger bones such as the femurs. If you are aching all over and feel like a ninety year old, then you probably have bone pain. I found Ibuprofen (consult your doctor before taking) very helpful in relieving the pain. If you are capable of going for a walk, it is a great way to help relieve and get your mind off the pain. Also a hot bath works.

Dear Caregiver: Bone pain can make your loved one very grumpy. It is very unpleasant and can last a few days.

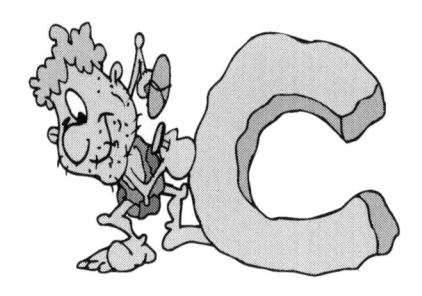

**Cancer**: a word, which we all wish, didn't exist. If I had the power I would annihilate that word and it's manifestations forever from our human existence. Unfortunately once you have been given the cancer label your life will never be the same. I have seen cancer destroy people and I have seen it create beautiful new people who continue their lives with a new purpose and an incredible will to live and make the most out of their days. We cannot know how cancer will affect us I can only suggest that you try your best during this worst of times to be positive and get through every day with dignity. Many doctors have told me that a patient's attitude can make a huge difference in their overall survival rate and experience. So let us all put our best foot forward and try to beat this disease if not physically, certainly mentally.

"You have cancer." Those three little words are fully loaded and not much else in this world evokes such strong emotions. How do you deal with this? Everyone may need help at some point in his or her journey. A good counselor or psychologist can really make a huge difference. Don't be afraid to ask for help. If you find a counselor and you don't feel better or right about it or the sessions don't leave you feeling heard then find someone else. Counseling if very personal and you need to have a good, therapeutic relationship for it to work.

Dear Caregiver: I understand your pain in having your loved one diagnosed with cancer. You are probably feeling powerless, hurt and angry. Your journey will also be a difficult one as you watch your friend, sister, and lover, go through their treatment. Please be kind to yourself and realize that you need a break too. Yours is in some ways a more challenging time because you aren't getting all the support that your loved one is. If you are open to counselling there is lots of individual and group support available to you. Just ask at your local cancer agency. Although your loved one may never express it, your help is invaluable to them. We cannot go through this without you. So here is a big Thank You to all caregivers. Please do not give up on us.

**Chemotherapy**: I could call this the worst hell you will ever go through, but that wouldn't be accurate because not all chemo will have you on your knees begging for it to end. I have written about some of the chemo drugs separately but there are so many chemo drugs available and thankfully I haven't experienced them so cannot discuss the way they make you feel. Suffice to say chemo is not fun and it will basically poison your entire body so you will feel sick as a dog and wish you never had to go to another chemo session again. As the days to the next session get closer, somehow you will get braver and your terrible memories of the past ones will start to fade and you will do it again, and again and as many times as you and your doctor feel you can handle it, all in an effort to kill this cancer and come out a survivor and fighter on the other side.

# THE CANCER WARRIOR HANDBOOK

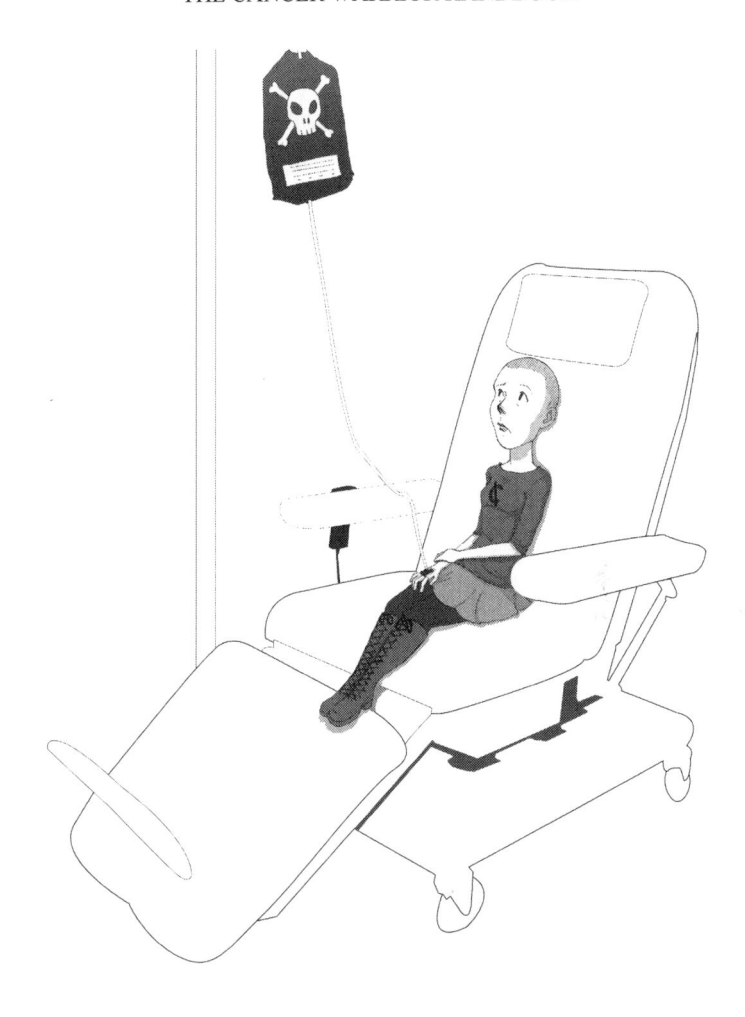

Now this looks really nasty. I wonder if I can run and hide.

**Constipation**: as if you don't have enough to deal with, now you can't go to the bathroom. There are few things more painful than trying to go to the bathroom after a few days of storing things up inside you. So, do your best to not let it get that far. I found drinking lots of fluids the two days before chemo and the days following really helped. Also make sure you get some natural roughage. If you still aren't able to go, ask your chemo nurse if you can take a gentle stool softener along with lots more water. Unfortunately I found that my constipation would lead to a few days of diarrhea then back to constipation until I learned to get it under control by starting my water regime before chemo.

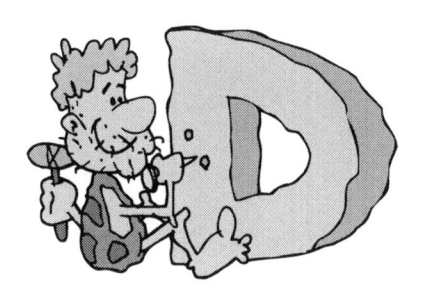

**Dexamethasone**: this drug made me go postal. I hated it; unfortunately it is one of the most common medications given when you go through chemo. From a purely technical point of view, Dexamethasone is a potent synthetic member of the glucocorticoid class of steroid drugs that has anti-inflammatory and immunosuppressant properties. It is twenty-five times more potent than cortisol in its glucocorticoid effect, while having minimal mineralocorticoid effect. Blah blah blah, basically it can make you nuts, but it is necessary to stop skin rash and some of the other chemo side effects. If you find the drug too challenging for you, speak to your oncologist about making some changes. I was able to reduce my daily intake after day one, and my oncologist completely changed my chemo regime after my A/C treatment so I wouldn't have to take as many steroids.

Dear Caregiver: this drug may turn your partner into a serious doer. They may start cleaning the house like crazy, organizing their office or the garage or be up all night working on projects. Enjoy it while it lasts.

**Diarrhea**: this can be never ending or can sway back and forth with constipation. After my chemo I found days one through three I was as constipated as a mule and days three through five were like a running river. This can get very painful not to mention being a pain in the ass. Chemo can cause changes in the lining of your whole digestive system. Cancer in your digestive system can cause bowel issues.

You never know when it is going to hit. Be prepared. Always know where the washrooms are and if needed, wear a small incontinence product. It's good to carry Imodium around. If this is not enough, ask your doctor for something stronger. Keep hydrated and take probiotics in your food or as a supplement. You also might need some type of cream to stop the pain around your anus. Talk to your doctor about what will work for you.

**Docetaxel**: also known as Taxotere. A chemotherapy drug typically administered at three-week intervals. A large amount of steroids are administered both before and after this drug in order to manage any adverse reactions. If you haven't already lost your hair from other chemotherapy agent, then you probably will from this drug. In some patients this drug can cause severe peripheral neuropathy (nerve damage that affects fingers and toes). Most cancer agencies will put ice-gloves and ice-booties on the patient during the treatment to help decrease the chances of the neuropathy. The good news is that over time this neuropathy should improve and in most cases will heal completely.

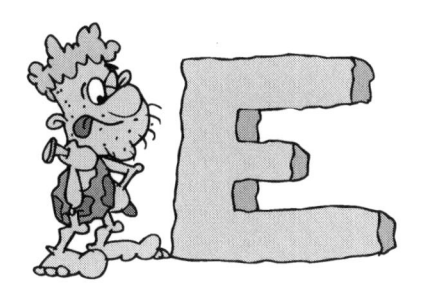

**Exhaustion**: described as a subjective feeling of tiredness. I can tell you, if you were going through chemo and radiation, you would not use the term tiredness. This can be so debilitating you can barely move and may find yourself sleeping for hours on end. I thought I had experienced exhaustion during chemotherapy, however it was radiation that really kicked me to the curb. They call it radiation fatigue. I call it radiation wipe out. Seriously, you will feel completely depleted and wiped out. It is quite normal; however if you are concerned, consult your radiation oncologist.

Dear Caregiver: now is the time when your loved one will require, sleep, sleep and more sleep. Make sure he or she is kept hydrated and continues to eat healthy meals. Good healthy food will help. No burgers or heavy junk food, that will just add to the feeling of exhaustion.

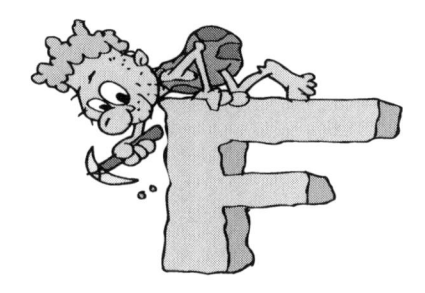

**Fatigue**: it seems everybody experiences fatigue. Treatments, the cancer and the stress all contribute. You can have time when it's hard to stay vertical and the couch is calling your name. You need to respect fatigue but don't let it get the best of you. This may sound contradictory but getting a bit of exercise can reduce fatigue. Prioritize, pace, conserve energy, ask for help, and keep a routine if possible. I found it best to get up and go for a little walk or bike ride first thing in the morning while I still had the energy. It pepped me up for the rest of the day.


**Finances**: hold on to your hat. Getting cancer is a very expensive proposition. Not only will you have lost your own income from being unable to work, but also it is also possible that your caregiver has had to reduce their work hours in order to look after you. You may also have expenses associated with drugs that aren't covered, vehicle and parking costs associated with driving for daily radiation or weekly chemo. Perhaps you have to stay in a city for a few weeks for treatment? Maybe you have to hire a caregiver? If you are having trouble getting a drug covered, try giving the drug company a call. They often have staff that will help you to get it covered, or a program where they will pay for it. Your local cancer agency may also be able to assist you with getting funding.


**Flamazine:** Silver sulfadiazine belongs to the class of medications called topical antibiotics. It is used to treat and prevent infection of skin wounds, especially in victims of serious burns. It may also be used in leg ulcers, skin grafts, surgical incisions, and minor cuts and scrapes. It is applied directly to the wounded area and works by stopping the action of bacteria that may cause infection. This may be prescribed to you to help treat burns from radiation therapy.

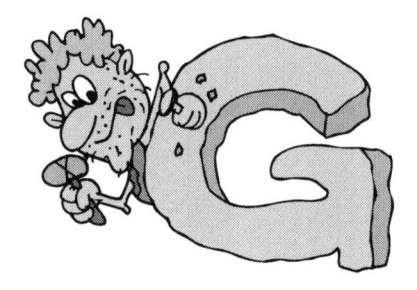

**Gefinitib:** also known as Iressa is used for certain breast and lung cancers. It can cause skin rashes, nausea, diarrhea and vomiting. In most cases this can be managed with the pre and post meds your oncologist will give you.

**Gemcitabine (Gemzar):** is a general use drug used for breast, pancreatic, lung and bladder cancer. It is a white powder that is then made up into a colourless liquid, administered intravenously and most often used to treat non-small cell lung cancer. It is generally quite well tolerated and is considered a lower toxicity chemotherapy agent.

Side effects can include: anemia and fatigue, a weakened immune system. You may get mouth ulcers, and a rash on your skin and it can temporarily affect the liver and kidneys.

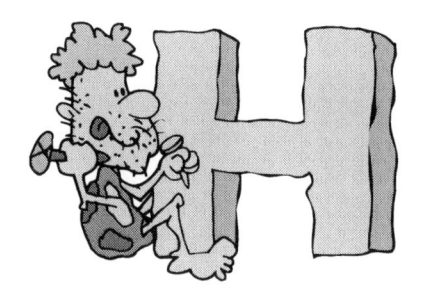

**Hair loss**: unfortunately this will affect almost everyone undergoing heavy chemotherapy. It only hurts a little; actually, mostly it hurts the ego. So if you can, get yourself some funky hats, bandanas or splurge on a wig. Eventually your hair will grow back even if it comes in grey and curly, it is better than having no hair at all. It is a good idea to get your hair cut very short before it starts falling out. It can be very heartbreaking to see large junks of hair on the pillow. It is also not so nice on the shower drain. So, take the bull by the horns and go and get a close-cropped cut, keep this for a week or two, but when the junks start falling out, just get your hairdresser to do the complete shave. Some folks even tattoo their bald heads. So be creative and enjoy your few months of looking like a cue ball. Most cancer agencies have second hand wigs you can borrow if your budget is tight and you really can't imagine wearing a scarf or bandana.

**Herceptin**: also known as Trastuzumab is a monoclonal antibody used to treat HER2 positive breast cancers. This drug is administered intravenously every three weeks. In terms of side affects, the Herceptin was no problem for me and is typically tolerated well by most patients. The biggest issue with Herceptin is that it can cause damage to the heart. In order to monitor this you will be getting regular Echo Cardio Gram's to look at the health of your heart. Your oncologist will stop the Herceptin if there appears to be any significant heart damage. Some patients may be on Herceptin for life, some for only a year. This is a very good drug for targeting HER2 positive cancers and has saved many lives.

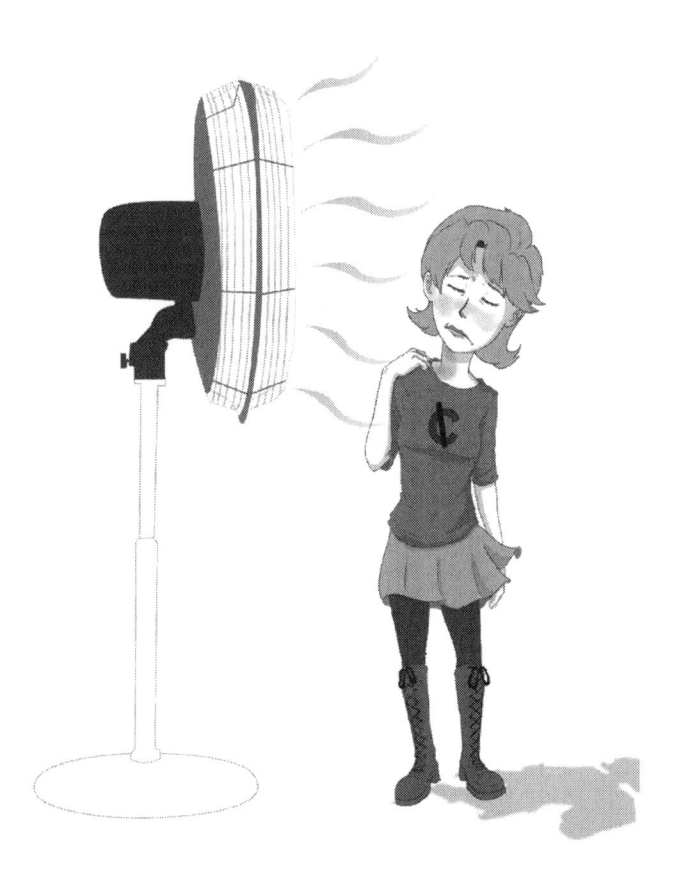

Can't you see I'm burning up?  Bring on the Firemen.

**Hot Flashes**:  oh my I could go on about these ad nauseam. Chemotherapy will throw your body into menopause (women only of course) if you have not already been there. The menopause type symptoms are more intense and shorter lived than when experiencing normal menopause. The hot flashes will come on so fast you will want to strip down to nothing, so be careful to wear layers when you go out in public. There is really no treatment for this other than to be aware that it will happen, use a cold compress on your forehead if you can get one in time, and just bear with it. It will be over soon and you will find yourself reaching for a blanket.

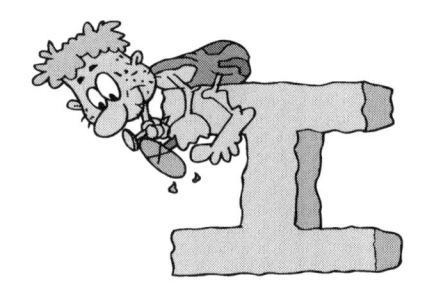

**Insomnia**: I have always slept on average ten to twelve hours a night. I know, this isn't the norm, but for me it has always been needed and I'm much happier when I get the proper amount of sleep. From my very first chemotherapy treatment until today (thirteen months later), I have been struggling with sleep. The Steroids they pre-medicated me with before the chemo added to the problem. In the beginning I would be lucky if I got five hours sleep a night and that was very broken, hot, sweaty and restless sleep. I used sleeping aids from the first month of chemo until about a month ago. One thing most oncologists will tell you is that you need your rest to heal and not to worry about the fact that you need to take something to help you sleep. I had tried everything from meditation to hot milk and honey before I finally agreed to take the sleeping pills and I am very glad I did. Now if I have trouble sleeping I just listen to a bit of my audio book and I'm out like a light

You NEED sleep, that's when your body heals.

Have a solid bedtime routine; make it dark and cool and calming about an hour before you want to go to bed. Turn off all the "screens", read a book, listen to mellow music or meditate. Do what you need to in order to sleep.

**Insurance**: unfortunately if you didn't have insurance before you got sick, it will be too late now. It is still an important topic to bring up so that it can be shared with those who can still do something about it. There are four types of insurance policies that will help minimize the impact of a cancer diagnosis from a financial perspective.

The first is Critical Illness Insurance; this type of coverage will pay you a lump sum (say $100,000.00) if you are diagnosed with a Critical Illness. This money is yours to use as you see fit, whether it is to seek alternative treatment in another country, to spend on modifications to your home, or to simply enjoy, the choice is yours.

The second type of insurance is Disability Insurance. Disability Insurance can only be purchased if you are working. This insurance will pay you a monthly income should you become disabled and unable to work (cancer prevents you from working, so the insurance will pay out). Quite often you can have disability insurance included in your company group plan. If you don't, it should be considered as a private insurance plan.

The third type of insurance is Personal Health Insurance. This will cover all or a portion of the cost of the drugs needed to recover. Again, quite often this is something you already have through your employment, but can be purchased privately if you don't.

Finally there is Long Term Care insurance. This insurance will be paid to you if you are unable to perform any of the six acts of daily living (such as toileting, feeding, transferring etc.) without assistance. Long Term Care insurance must be purchased privately.

So, again, this may be too late for some of us, but good information to know to share with those we love.

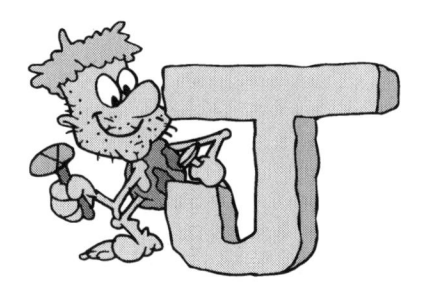

**Jitters, jumpiness**: with all the steroids you may have to take to offset the chemotherapy side effects, you will probably experience some degree of jitters. I don't mean the nervous jitters you get before every chemotherapy or radiation session. I mean a general uneasiness and shakiness in your body. Your heart may race and you may feel shortness of breath. Try sitting in a nice quiet place and do some deep breathing or meditation to help relax. In some cases, the racing heart and shortness of breath could mean something more serious like an allergic reaction to one of your drugs, so don't underestimate it. If the feeling of unease lasts more than a few minutes or gets worse, call your doctor or go to the clinic immediately.

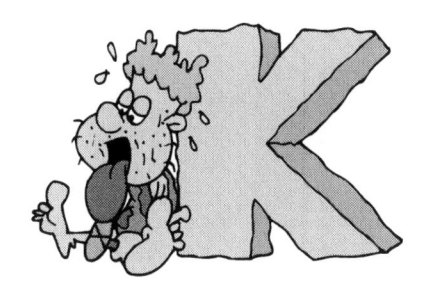

**Knowledge**: knowledge is a powerful tool when it comes to being a self-advocate and fighting your battle against cancer. Get as much information as you can about your disease and the best clinics that offer treatment as well as understanding the different treatment protocols. In the United States you can go to clinics in different states that may offer better treatment for your specific cancer. Do your research, but beware, not everything you read on the Internet is true, and in the beginning, too much of the wrong information can be overwhelming. Stay away from statistics. I know for some of you (like it was for me), the survival statistics of my disease was the first thing I wanted to know. Don't do it, unless of course you are one of the lucky ones with a ninety percent or more survival rate. I found the statistics would bring me down and being depressed and helpless about fighting cancer is not going to work. So ignore the statistics, everything is really individual so focus on the good stuff and your battle and that you will get through it.

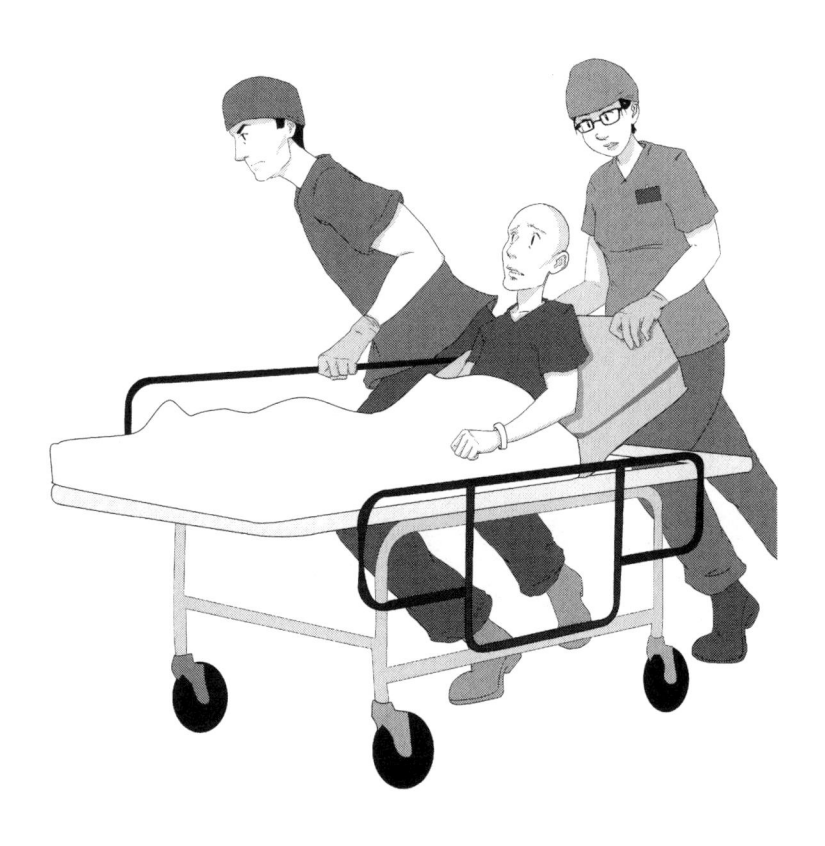

Just what the heck have I got myself into?

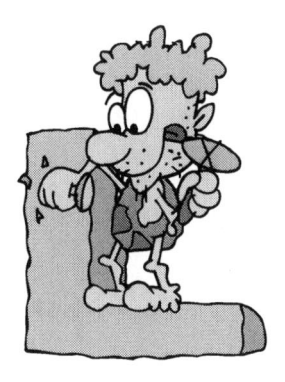

**Lemons and Lemon Juice**: maybe you've received the email about lemon juice (insert other new options here - soursop, DCA) being stronger than chemo and killing cancer cells. You've probably even heard that there is a conspiracy to suppress this information by the drug companies. Someone somewhere took cancer cells in a petri dish or test tube and made this claim. It could very well be true. But we don't actually know what happens inside the human body. Lemon juice alone will not likely cure you but it tastes pretty good, is healthy and it's affordable so you may as well add it to your diet. A wonderfully easy way to do this is to have hot (not boiling) water with lemon every morning upon awakening and before you have anything else to eat or drink. Here are ten of the benefits of drinking hot water and lemon every morning.

1) **Aids Digestion.** Lemon juice flushes out unwanted materials and toxins from the body. Its atomic composition is similar to saliva and the hydrochloric acid of digestive juices. It encourages the liver to produce bile, which is an acid that is required for digestion. Lemons are also high in minerals and vitamins and help loosen ama, or toxins, in the digestive tract. The digestive qualities of lemon juice help to relieve symptoms of indigestion, such as heartburn, belching and bloating. The American Cancer Society actually recommends offering warm lemon water to cancer sufferers to help stimulate bowel movements.

2) **Cleanses Your System / is a Diuretic.** Lemon juice helps flush out unwanted materials in part because lemons increase the rate of urination in the body. Therefore toxins are released at a

faster rate, which helps keep your urinary tract healthy. The citric acid in lemons helps maximize enzyme function, which stimulates the liver and aids in detoxification.

3) **Boosts Your Immune System.** Lemons are high in vitamin C, which is great for fighting colds. They're high in potassium, which stimulates brain and nerve function. Potassium also helps control blood pressure. Ascorbic acid (vitamin C) found in lemons demonstrates anti-inflammatory effects, and is used as complementary support for asthma and other respiratory symptoms plus it enhances iron absorption in the body; iron plays an important role in immune function. Lemons also contain saponins, which show antimicrobial properties that may help keep cold and flu at bay. Lemons also reduce the amount of phlegm produced by the body.

4) **Balances pH Levels**. Lemons are one of the most alkalizing foods for the body. Sure, they are acidic on their own, but inside our bodies they're alkaline (the citric acid does not create acidity in the body once metabolized). Lemons contain both citric and ascorbic acid, weak acids easily metabolized from the body allowing the mineral content of lemons to help alkalize the blood. Disease states only occur when the body pH is acidic. Drinking lemon water regularly can help to remove overall acidity in the body, including uric acid in the joints, which is one of the primary causes of pain and inflammation.

5) **Clears Skin.** The vitamin C component as well as other antioxidants helps decrease wrinkles and blemishes and it helps to combat free radical damage. Vitamin C is vital for healthy glowing skin while its alkaline nature kills some types of bacteria known to cause acne. It can actually be applied directly to scars or age spots to help reduce their appearance. Since lemon water purges toxins from your blood, it would also be helping to keep your skin clear of blemishes from the inside out. The vitamin C contained in the lemon rejuvenates the skin from within your body.

6) **Energizes You and Enhances Your Mood.** The energy a human receives from food comes from the atoms and molecules in your food. A reaction occurs when the positive charged ions from

food enter the digestive tract and interact with the negative charged enzymes. Lemon is one of the few foods that contain more negative charged ions, providing your body with more energy when it enters the digestive tract. The scent of lemon also has mood enhancing and energizing properties. The smell of lemon juice can brighten your mood and help clear your mind. Lemon can also help reduce anxiety and depression.

7) **Promotes Healing.** Ascorbic acid (vitamin C), found in abundance in lemons, promotes wound healing, and is an essential nutrient in the maintenance of healthy bones, connective tissue, and cartilage. As noted previously, vitamin C also displays anti-inflammatory properties. Combined, vitamin C is an essential nutrient in the maintenance of good health and recovery from stress and injury.

8) **Freshens Breath.** Besides fresher breath, lemons have been known to help relieve tooth pain and gingivitis. Be aware that citric acid can erode tooth enamel, so you should be mindful of this. Do not brush your teeth just after drinking your lemon water. It is best to brush your teeth first, then drink your lemon water, or wait a significant amount of time after to brush your teeth. Additionally, you can rinse your mouth with purified water after you finish your lemon water.

9) **Hydrates Your Lymph System.** Warm water and lemon juice supports the immune system by hydrating and replacing fluids lost by your body. When your body is deprived of water, you can definitely feel the side effects, which include: feeling tired, sluggish, decreased immune function, constipation, lack of energy, low/high blood pressure, lack of sleep, lack of mental clarity and feeling stressed, just to name a few.

10) **Aids in Weight Loss.** Lemons are high in pectin fiber, which helps fight hunger cravings. Studies have shown people who maintain a more alkaline diet, do in fact lose weight faster.

For more information you can read further at:
http://tasty-yummies.com/2013/03/18/10-benefits-to-drinking-warm-lemon-water-every-morning/

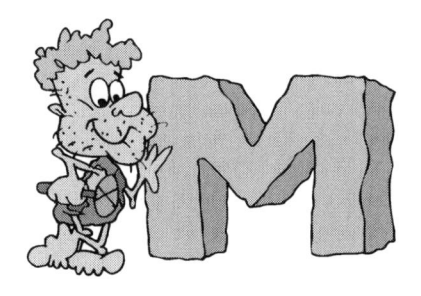

**Medical Marijuana**: I am not a pot smoker and was initially quite concerned by the suggestion to try marijuana to treat my nausea and other chemotherapy related symptoms. However, after a long conversation with my GP about the benefits of marijuana, not just for treating symptoms, but also for cancer prevention, I decided to give it a shot. As a non-smoker, I chose to consume my medical marijuana orally. In order to do this, one needs to get a membership and obtain the marijuana from a licensed medical marijuana distributor. I used drops diluted in a small amount of water as my preferred method. The results after my second chemotherapy session were amazing. I felt a hundred times better than I had the previous session and am positive it was due to the marijuana. It did not make me feel stoned or sleepy in any way (I was already sleepy from the other drugs I had to take following chemo), rather it simply eased the horrible nausea and gave me some peace.

The anti-nausea effects of medicinal marijuana are well known both scientifically and among users who have experienced **relief from nausea and vomiting**. While cannabinoids isolated from the cannabis plant also help to mitigate nausea, smoking medical marijuana provides superior treatment for vomiting when compared to THC ingested orally. THC also improved appetite and reduced weight loss in patients living with AIDS, as a 2007 study showed. In a similar study during the same year in which scientists surveyed HIV-positive marijuana smokers, both THC and medical marijuana resulted in an increase in caloric intake and in weight.

While synthetic THC in oral form provides some of the benefits of smoked medical marijuana, many patients prefer to smoke or vaporize cannabis instead of taking a THC pill. **Cannabis is a fully renewable resource and, depending upon local marijuana laws, patients may be permitted to grow medical marijuana at home rather than traveling to a pharmacy for their medication.** In 1991, 54% of clinical oncologists surveyed felt that their patients should be able to obtain medical marijuana by prescription for nausea and other symptoms.

Medical marijuana is even effective for some patients whose nausea does not respond to traditional antiemetic medications. In one study published in the New York State Journal of Medicine, fifty-six patients were treated whose nausea symptoms had not responded to traditional antiemetic drugs. Of these fifty-six patients, **78% saw improvement after smoking medical marijuana.**

For more information you can read further at:
http://www.medicalmarijuana.net/uses-and-treatments/nausea/

**Meditation**: before having cancer I can't say I ever meditated. I would sometimes use this technique I learned in drama class when I was a teenager to help me sleep at night. I suppose in a sense it was a form of meditation, however that was as far as I ever got. When I first got diagnosed I was understandably an emotional mess and kept most of that pain and sense of loss inside. I had to find a way to deal with it, so I decided to download some guided meditation onto my iPhone. I started with Louise L. Hay's book Cancer: Discovering Your Healing Power, then moved on to Esther and Jerry Hicks, The Law of Attraction: The Basics of the Teachings of Abraham and finally I got Deepak Chopra The Secret of Healing and Quantum Healing.

I cannot definitively say listening to these helped my body get rid of the cancer (along with the chemo, surgery and radiation), but I can say it made me feel better and helped me get through the tough days and nights.

Living the cancer journey is a wild roller coaster ride. You need to find a way to hold on and ride it without being thrown off. Meditation can be a great tool to use. There has even been a lot of great research on the mind's ability to help in the healing process.

Other than the audiobooks that I downloaded to my iPhone, there are library CD's, Podcasts and online streaming options for guided meditation that cost nothing. Most are non-denominational. Yoga studios often offer meditation sessions.

There is an eight-week program called the Mindfulness Based Stress Reduction program in which you learn the basics of Mindfulness Meditation. Most local cancer agencies put this on a few times a year. Google MBSR.

**Mouth Sores**: these can be horrible, but the mouthwash to treat them is even worse. Mouth sores are standard fare when on certain chemotherapy drugs. The sores can be anywhere in your mouth and even down your esophagus that is why the mouthwash you are given needs to be swirled and swallowed. It is disgusting and made me gag and almost vomit. However, it works like a charm and after a few treatments, the mouth sores were gone. As mouth sores can be such a pain, literally, here are a few helpful hints to try and prevent them:

- Clean your teeth or dentures gently every morning and evening.
- Use a soft-bristled or child's toothbrush. Toothbrush bristles can also be softened in hot water. An electric toothbrush can clean your teeth very effectively.
- Replace your toothbrush frequently to prevent problems with infection.
- If your toothpaste stings, you could try using a non-foaming toothpaste. Ask your specialist nurse to advise you on the best one to use.
- If brushing your teeth makes you feel sick, use a saline (salty water) mouthwash four times a day. (Make it by

adding 1 teaspoon of salt to 1 pint of cold or warm water.) After using the mouthwash, rinse your mouth with cold or warm water.

- If you've been sick, rinse out your mouth before cleaning your teeth, as the acid in your vomit may damage your teeth.
- If your doctor or nurse prescribes a mouthwash for you, use it regularly as prescribed.
- You can gently use dental tape or floss daily, but check with your doctor or nurse first. Dental flossing should be avoided if the level of platelets in your blood is low (called thrombocytopenia), or if you're having radiotherapy to the head or neck area. This is because a low platelet count can cause bleeding in the mouth, even with very gentle flossing. Toothpicks should not be used.
- Keep your lips moist by using Vaseline®, or a lip balm if you prefer. If you're having radiotherapy to your head or neck area, check with your radiotherapy team or specialist nurse before using these products on your lips.
- Avoid alcohol, tobacco, hot spices, (I know and I said I put Franks Red Hot on everything) garlic, onion, vinegar and salty foods, as these may irritate your mouth.
- Some crunchy foods may damage your gums and should be avoided when your white blood cell counts are low.
- Keep your mouth and food moist. Add gravies and sauces to your food to help with swallowing.
- If you're finding it difficult to eat because your mouth is sore, ask your doctor, nurse or a dietitian for advice about taking food supplements. Your doctor or nurse can prescribe some supplements.
- Try to drink at least 1.5 litres (3 pints) of fluid a day. This can include water, tea, weak coffee, and soft drinks such as apple juice.
- Avoid acidic drinks, such as orange or grapefruit juice. Warm herbal teas may be more soothing.
- Let your doctor or nurse know if you have mouth ulcers, as you may need medicines to help heal the ulcers and clear infection.

MacMillan Cancer Support provided the above tips. For more information you can go to their website at: http://www.macmillan.org.uk/Cancerinformation/Livingwithandaftercancer/Symptomssideeffects/Mouthcare/Chemotherapy.aspx

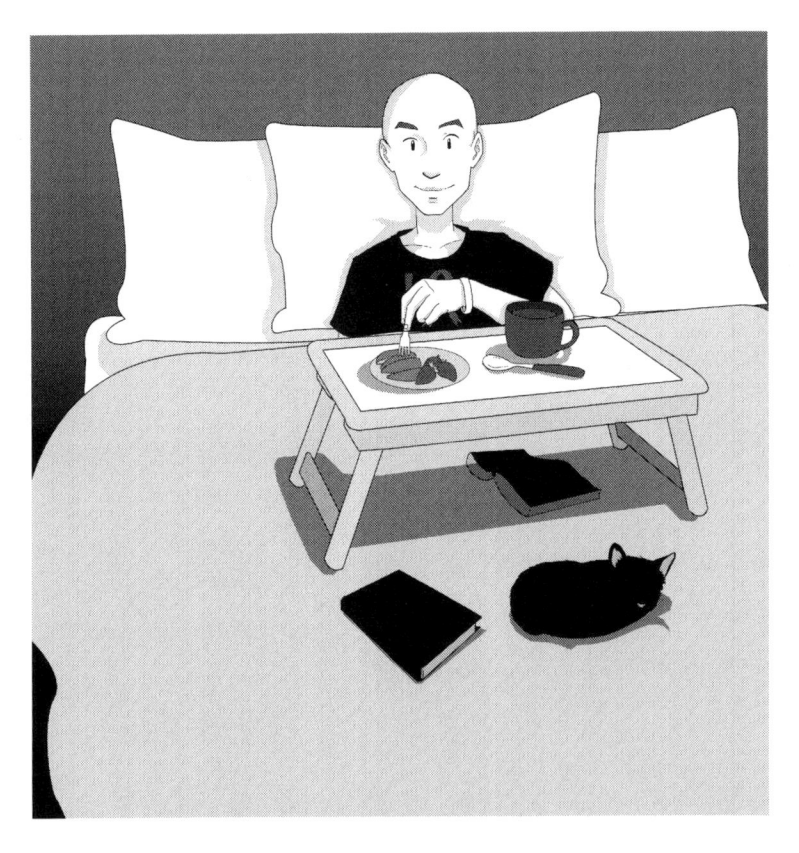

You want me to eat? My mouth tastes like a metal factory.

**Music**: hands down, music can be one of the most powerful tools in healing, grieving, celebrating and remaining joyous. Music can be used as a tool to help you dig deep into your grief and pain and bring it out to the surface so that you can heal. I start off my day with a hot shower and some great upbeat music. No matter how I feel when I step out of bed, I always feel happy and ready to face my day after my shower and dancing tunes. Every cancer warrior needs a kick ass playlist and maybe an introspective one. Music can be energy lifting, soothing, creative, and healing. Find the kind of music you love and play it as much as possible. Just be careful not to focus solely on sad, depressing music, you don't want to get to a place that will be hard to get back up from.

Dear Caregiver; if you see your loved one bawling over a song or dancing like crazy in the shower, don't fret, they are only just a little nuts but will come out of it.

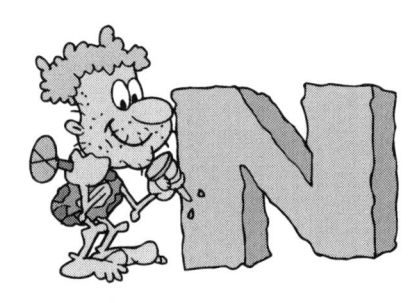

**Neuropathy**: is damage to nerves of the peripheral nervous system, which may be caused either by diseases of or trauma to the nerve or the side effects of systemic illness. Some chemo drugs such as Taxol (Paclitaxel) can cause neuropathy in the fingers and toes (peripheral neuropathy). You could experience a numbness of tingling in the hands or feet. In some rare cases it can be painful. For me I found it frustrating because I lost my fine motor skills for a short while and typing was almost impossible. Almost all cases of neuropathy caused by chemotherapy will disappear over time, but it does take time. It has been eight months since my last Taxol treatment and my toenails are still falling out and the fingernails are full of ridges. Nothing a good manicure or pedicure can't take care of temporarily. Hey, who says guys can't get a manicure? If that's not your bag, keep your nails short and clean to minimize breakage. You can even ask your chemo nurse if it is possible to use icepacks on your hands and feed during the administration of the Taxol or Taxotere. This will lessen the neuropathy.


**Nutrition**: we all know super healthy people - raw, vegan, all organic - that get cancer and fast food eating smokers that don't get cancer. Refer to hundreds of thousands, maybe millions of books, articles and Internet resources on the topic. Beware of the guilt and blame conspiracy theories. Find what resonates with you and helps you heal. Don't beat yourself up.

Best advice I've received: eat real, unprocessed food in its whole form, mostly plants and don't overeat. The odd piece of chocolate or order of fries is not going to singularly cause your cancer to return.

Listen to your body - what is it asking for you to eat. You'd be surprised at how your body asks for healthy options if you are listening.

**Nausea**: quite frankly nausea sucks. For chemo related nausea, they have some pretty amazing new medications. You take these before and after treatment on a tight schedule often along with some steroids. These all work together to control nausea.

You have to stay on top of nausea. The second you start to feel unwell, take your meds. If you wait too long you will be hugging the porcelain throne or in the hospital on IV.

Sometimes the drugs they give you for nausea do not work for you. Let your doctor know, as there are many other drugs they can try.

Nausea and vomiting, whether due to chemotherapy, radiation, or another cause, can be effectively remedied through the use of medical marijuana. Clinical trials and patients' experiences indicate that smoking or ingesting medical marijuana can both relieve nausea and stimulate the appetites of patients with nausea, reducing the risk of unhealthy weight loss in patients. (See the section on Medical Marijuana for more information)

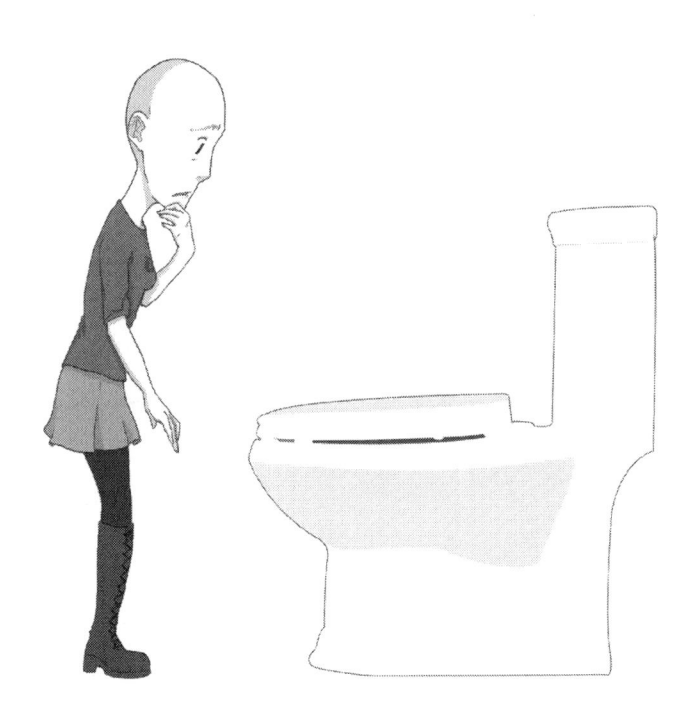

Hello old friend.  Here we go again.

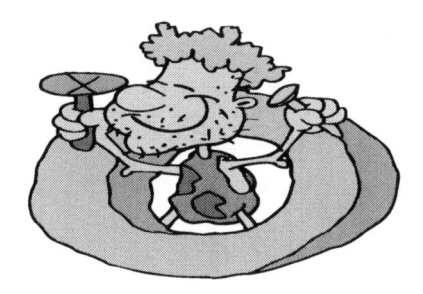

**Orgasms**: having cancer can kill your sex drive. It starts with the ravages of chemo, and then you don't feel sexy because you've lost all your hair, or perhaps getting an erection is challenging, or you have been thrown into menopause. There can be many causes for loss of sex drive and lack of sensation during your cancer treatment. Rest assured, slowly things will return to normal. It can take up to a year and a half after all your treatments are complete, but in most cases you will get your sex drive back and be able to function normally again. If you are really struggling, go and see your family doctor. He or she will have some solutions for you to bring things back a little quicker.

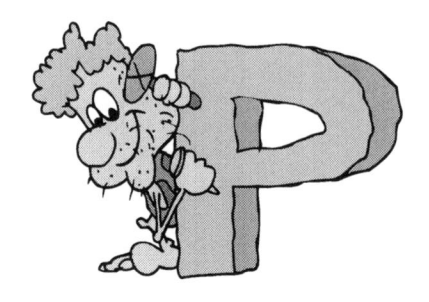

**Pain**: tumour pain, bone pain, nerve pain, muscle pain, joint pain, surgical pain, the pain come in many shapes and sizes. YOU DON'T NEED TO SUFFER. If you stay on top of pain, it won't overwhelm you. When you wait until it's unbearable, it takes longer and stronger medications to manage it. Keep a journal of your pain levels on a scale of 1-10 and write down what you take or what you do (breathing, massage, etc.) and how much. It gets pretty blurry at times and this helps your team come up with a plan.

When used for pain, narcotics and other strong medications will not make you addicted. It's when you start using them recreationally that it is a problem. Always check with your doctor before taking any pain medication to make sure it is correct for you. Remember this book is a guide, we are not making any recommendations regarding whether or not you take pain medication. That is a conversation between you and your physician.

**Pets**: I thank my wonderful dog Waldo for helping me get through some of my very dark days. Animals are amazing creatures and they seem to know when you need them most. Waldo lay by my side constantly when I was going through chemo and radiation. The hard part was having him understand how sore my body was after surgery and that he could not put his head on my lap for quite a while. If you have an animal you love, they will be of great comfort during this time.

They say that having a pet increases your likelihood of survival. I am not sure how accurate that is, but pets can definitely improve your quality of life. Caring for a pet gives you a reason to get up, walk, exercise, feed and groom. Pets can give you unconditional love and affection. They can lick all your tears and snuggle your fears away.

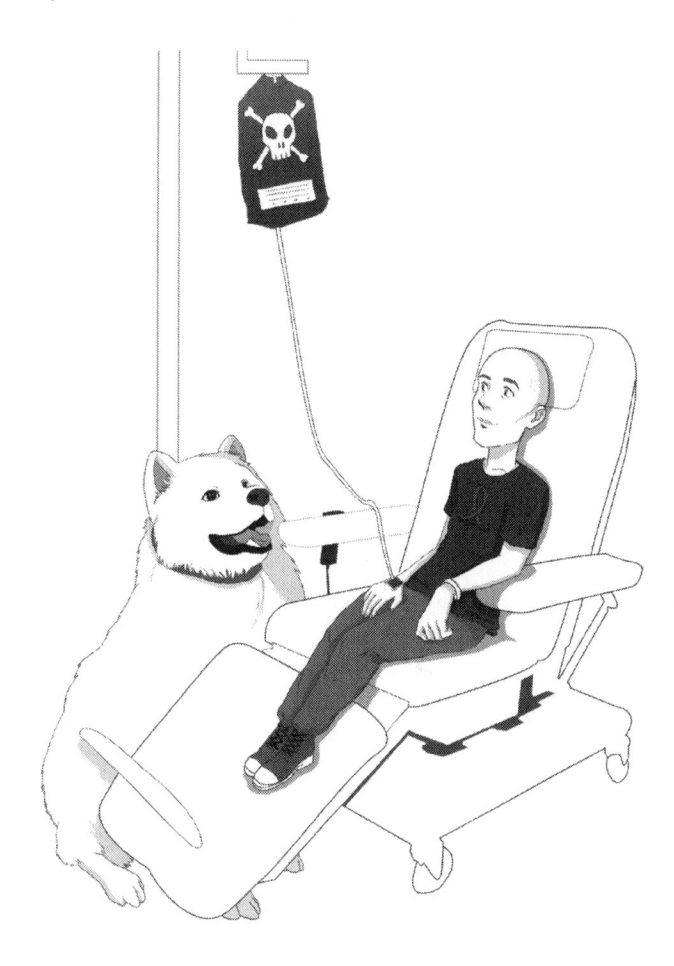

True Love.

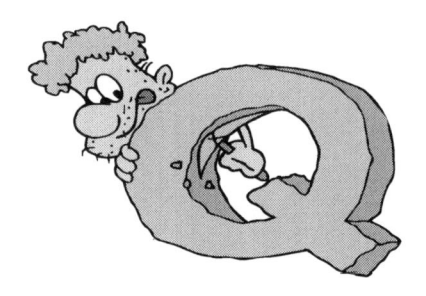

**Questions**: if you are like me, you will have a long list of questions when you first see your oncologist. Write them all down and make sure you write down the answers, as chemo brain will make you forget. I found the more I knew, the better I felt and the more I felt I was in control of my treatment program. It also helps to ask others who are going through, or went through the same treatments that you are. Don't feel embarrassed to ask anything, it has probably been asked before.

Dear Caregiver: you will no doubt have a lot of questions as well. It is important for you to get some answers. Your job over the next little while is to be there for your loved one both physically and emotionally. In order to do that successfully, you need to have some knowledge about the disease and what things may come up for you. So ask away and if things aren't clear, ask someone else or look it up on line or at your public library. You may also want to attend a weekly support group for caregivers. This can be a huge source of information and help for you.

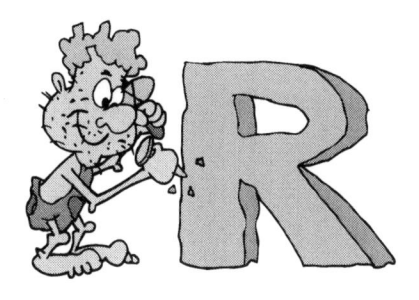

**Radiation**: I had a real issue with radiation. The whole idea of deliberately submitting my body to radiation (something that is poisonous and known to kill) was completely insane to me. I know they claim the amount of radiation they give you to treat your cancer is manageable and that it won't kill you, but really if they did that amount on a large portion of your body, then yes, it would kill you, or at the very least, it would cause cancer. So for me I had a big mental block when it came to radiation. From a purely clinical standpoint, Radiation therapy may be curative in a number of types of cancer if they are localized to one area of the body. It may also be used as part of adjuvant therapy, to prevent tumor recurrence after surgery to remove a primary malignant tumor (for example, early stages of breast cancer). Radiation therapy is synergistic with chemotherapy, and has been used before, during, and after chemotherapy in susceptible cancers. You can have Total Body Radiation (TBI) to prepare the body to receive a bone marrow transplant, Brachytherapy, in which a radiation source is placed inside or next to the area requiring treatment, standard radiation and radiation involving the use of a bolus (gel pack applied to the skin to deliberately burn the skin tissue). The longer the treatment, the worse the pain and side affects will be. I have spoken to people who had no skin burning at all, and then I've seen examples of people whose entire radiated area is blistered and burned. In my case I had to have a bolus applied for each treatment so my skin started showing signs of burning by about the fifth day. Rest assured, the nurses in the radiation facility are amazing. They will apply cooling saline compresses after each treatment to help with the cooking and burning of your flesh. They can arrange for a prescription of Flamazine (see details under Flamazine), for helping the skin to feel better. If things get really bad, they can arrange for the radiation oncologist to write you a prescription for painkillers. Between that and wine I found I could manage somewhat and forced myself through the twenty-eight days of hell.

**Radioactivity**: between radiation and nuclear scans you will definitely have your dose of radioactivity. Perhaps you will get some superpowers from it such as flying, reading minds, fortune telling perhaps. The ability to self repair and heal would be a nice bonus. Being radiated can make you feel sick and exhausted. It is a good idea to keep hydrated, if the nausea gets too bad; speak to your doctor about what you can take to help stop it. You may be warned to stay away from adolescents and young children, or if your treatment is really strong, you may have to be in isolation in the hospital. This will improve over time. On the bright side, at least you will glow if you go through security at the airport.

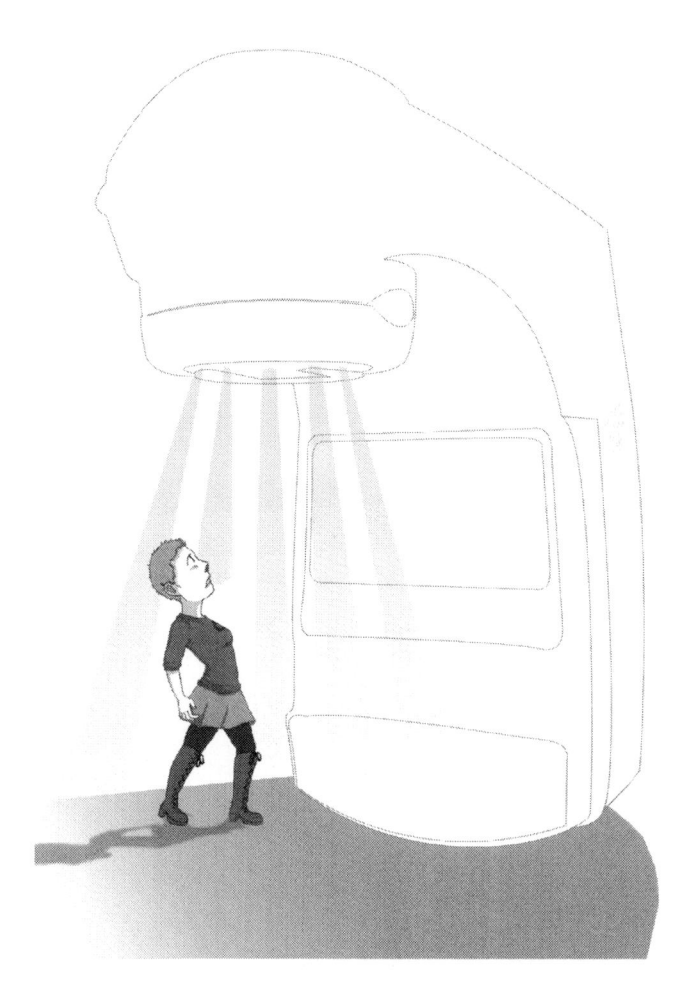

Beam me up Scotty.

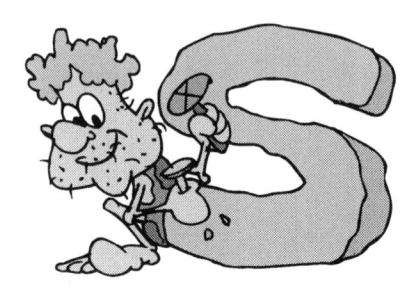

**Smart phone apps:** thank goodness will live in such a modern day and age and we can spend our time waiting for treatment or doctors appointments play apps on our smart phones. Instead of being nervous about your upcoming scan, or frustrated that your oncologist is running late again, pull out that phone and play a game of Temple Run or Angry Birds. The time will pass quickly and you will feel much less angst.


**Sex Drive**: what is that? Only kidding. Yes, having cancer can kill your sex drive. Really, who feels sexy when they have lost all their hair, their body is pumped with chemicals and they may have had body parts removed. Don't worry though, it will get better, you will enjoy sex again, just give it time. (Read the section under Orgasms for more information).

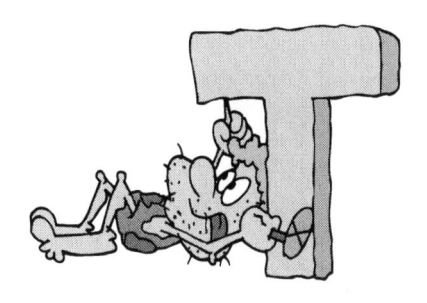

**Taste Changes**: otherwise known as metal mouth. Chemotherapy and radiation can both destroy your ability to taste food properly. In almost all cases this is temporary, but it sucks. Most food will taste like metal or completely bland. My solution was to eat food that had a strong or unique flavor - a favourite being pineapple and cottage cheese, or to add extra flavour to my food. Throughout chemo I was addicted to Franks Red Hot sauce. I added it to everything. Except of course my pineapple and cottage cheese.

I was told not to eat my favourite foods during chemo, as I would hate them when I was finished. Fortunately this did not happen to me, but if you are sensitive to food smells and tastes, you might want to avoid something you love for the time being. What I did find interesting was that cooked food did not appeal to me within the first few days after my chemo treatment. Fresh tropical fruit, cold Haagen Dazs ice cream and smoothies were the way to go.

Experiment a bit; you will eventually find what works for you. It is important to keep eating well as the chemo is sucking all your energy out of you. In the end, when you get your taste buds back you will be so thrilled at how great food tastes and will barely remember the terrible metal mouth days.

**Trust**: when you are dealing with the initial chaos of a cancer diagnosis, and then the healing process, you need to trust your healing team. Compassion, empathy, hopefulness and caring go a long way in increasing your chances to heal. Whether it's your oncologist, naturopath, shamanic healer or chemo nurse you NEED to feel a level of trust. But you also have to deal with your team in the same manner - treat others the way you wish to be treated. If you are not comfortable with your healer, you always have a right to a second and third and fourth opinion.

In today's world you really need to be your own advocate when it comes to navigating the medical system. If something seems wrong to you then question it. Do not stop until you get an answer you are satisfied with. In the long run the doctors are trying to do their best, but you know your body better than anyone, so listen to it and follow your instincts.

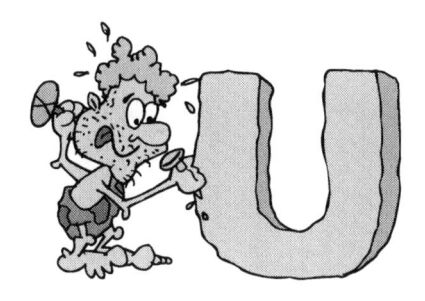

**Understanding**:  be kind to yourself and give yourself a little slack during this tough time.  This could possibly be the hardest few months of your life, so you will not be able to do things you normally do.  Understand and accept that.  Love yourself, take care of yourself and realize the value in the little achievements.  If you cannot get out of bed until noon, so be it, but when you do get up, have a nice shower, go for a short walk, or get outside to enjoy nature.  Remember, you are still alive on this wonderful planet. Keep putting one foot in front of the other and one day this will all be over.

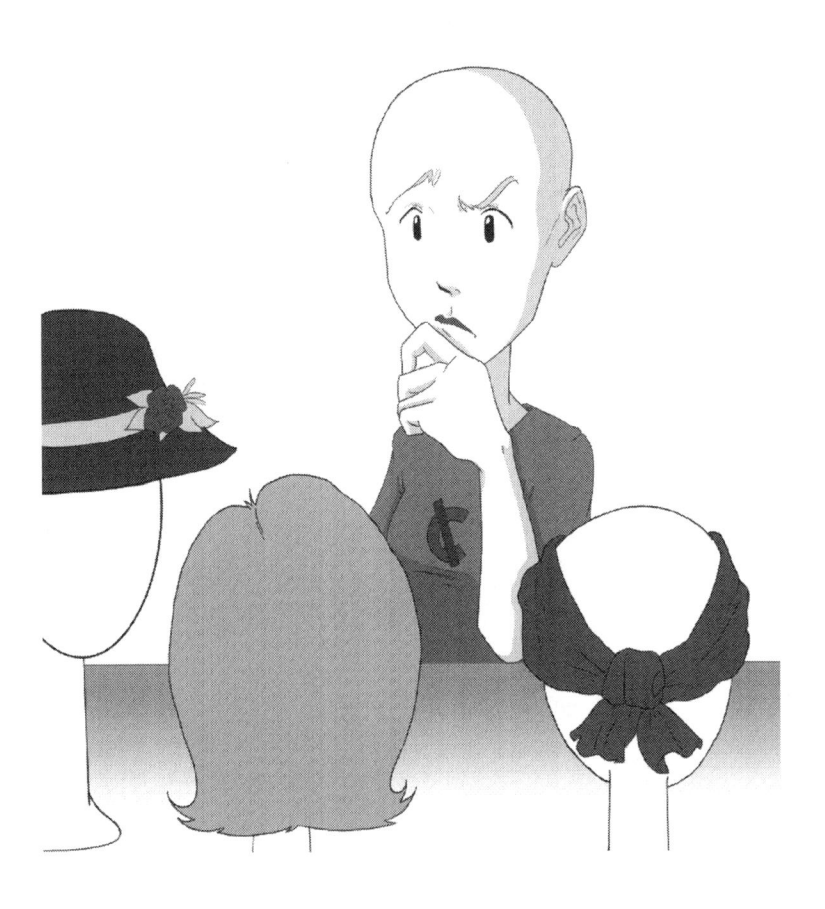

So many choices.  How is a girl to decide?

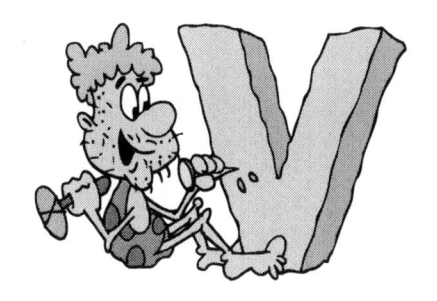

**Vomiting**: unfortunately vomiting is a major side effect of chemotherapy and in some cases radiation. This is not only horrible to live through, but can be very dangerous if you are not keeping your food and fluids down. Vomiting can make you dehydrated and is hard on your body. A few suggestions to prevent this from happening are to get on top of it early. Take your chemo pre and post nausea meds. If they don't work for you, speak to your doctor about stronger ones. Consider medical marijuana, which can be a great anti-nausea treatment. Stay hydrated as much as you can, even if you can only suck on ice-chips. Your body needs liquid and especially to help it flush out all the horrible medications you have been injected with.

Dear caregiver; please remember to wear gloves when cleaning up after your loved one. The toxins from the chemotherapy can be in any bodily fluid, so protect yourself.

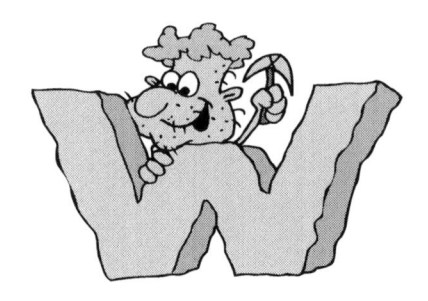

**Water Retention**: certain drugs can cause water retention. It may not seem like much in the beginning, but if your hands and feet get really swollen it can actually hurt. Fluid retention occurs when your body cannot remove fluid from the tissues as easily as usual, so the fluid builds up making the area puffy and sore. Other than the drugs, there are other things that can cause fluid retention, such as heart, liver or kidney failure. If you find you have fluid retention that lasts more than a day or so, or builds up to your ankles and your legs, consult your doctor immediately. They will check to ensure it is nothing serious, and may be able to prescribe something to take the swelling down.


**Weight Changes**: almost everyone will experience some type of weight change during their battle with cancer. The changes can be brought on by the cancer itself, or by the drugs used to treat the cancer, or by loss of appetite caused by either the drugs or the cancer. When you go for your chemo treatments, they will ask you to weigh yourself before each treatment. There are two reasons for this. The first is to know the exact amount of medication to mix for your body weight, but more importantly is the second reason, which is to ensure you are not loosing or gaining too much weight. Loosing too much weight during treatment is hard on your body and weakens your body's ability to fight the disease. Gaining too much weight can be a sign that something else is going on, perhaps the treatment protocol is wrong for you or perhaps something else is happening within your body. If you are on a lot of steroids, you will gain some weight, and your oncologist will let you know what is normal so make sure you discuss this with him or her. I lost about ten pounds throughout my cancer treatment, and of course this thrills me, however, it did present a problem when it came to my surgery because I didn't have enough abdominal fat and was almost not able to have the procedure. Thanks to Haagen Dazs every evening I managed to squeak by.

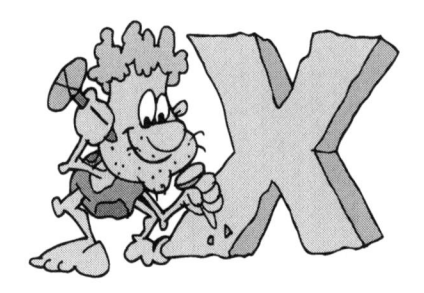

**X-ray's (Dental)**: chemotherapy kills cancer cells, but it also kills healthy cells, including the ones in your mouth. It can affect your gums, your saliva and the lining of your mouth. You need to watch for infection, as that can be dangerous when you are on chemo. Try to get a dental check up before your start your treatment if you have an opportunity to. However, if you do need to see your dentist because of teeth, gum or mouth issues, and he recommends a dental x-ray, don't be concerned. Having an x-ray during chemo will be just fine. Your dentist probably won't recommend any treatment until after you are done your chemotherapy, as the risk of infection is too great.

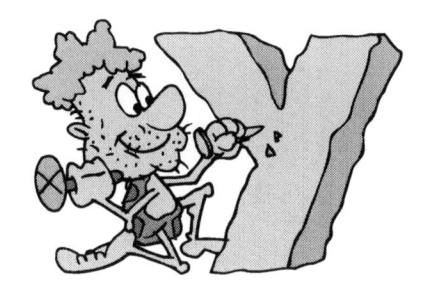

**Yoga**: the only yoga I did prior to getting cancer was P90X yoga (which was pure hell), and a daily yoga app that was on my iPhone. I'm too impatient for yoga, I know, that is the point, yoga is meant to help me relax, but I find it stressful, so didn't do too much of it during my illness other than the limited yoga we did at one of my healing retreats.

All this being said, most people find yoga to be a terrific healing tool so perhaps yoga it will be part of your healing journey. Many cancer warriors choose take this path. There are poses made just for us - Warrior 1, Warrior 2 and so on. It's more than just exercise. It is a very mindful and meditative activity so the mental benefits abound. If you are weak, tired and unable to handle strenuous activity, try a Restorative or Yin class.

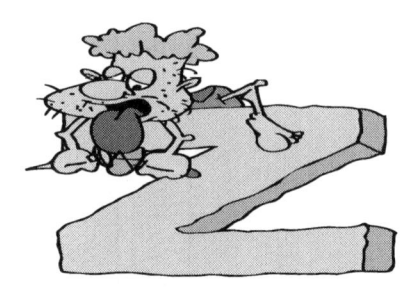

**Zopiclone**: the reason for my sanity throughout my treatment. Zopiclone also known as Imovane is used to treat insomnia. I did not take sleeping pills prior to getting sick and initially had a huge issue with it, but as my oncologist said. Taking sleeping pills in moderation is better than getting no sleep at all. We need the sleep to heal and fight the disease. I found Zopiclone to be a good solution, however it typically only worked for about five hours, and it does leave an awful taste in your mouth. Remember; consult your doctor to see Zopiclone could be right for you. After prolonged use, your body can become accustomed to the drug. Stopping or reducing the drug after a long period of use can cause withdrawal symptoms and chronic nightly use can cause daytime anxiety. So once again, ensure this is the right drug for you by checking with your doctor. For me it was a life saver and now that my treatment regime is over I find I no longer need it and have slowly returned to a normal sleep pattern without the drugs help.

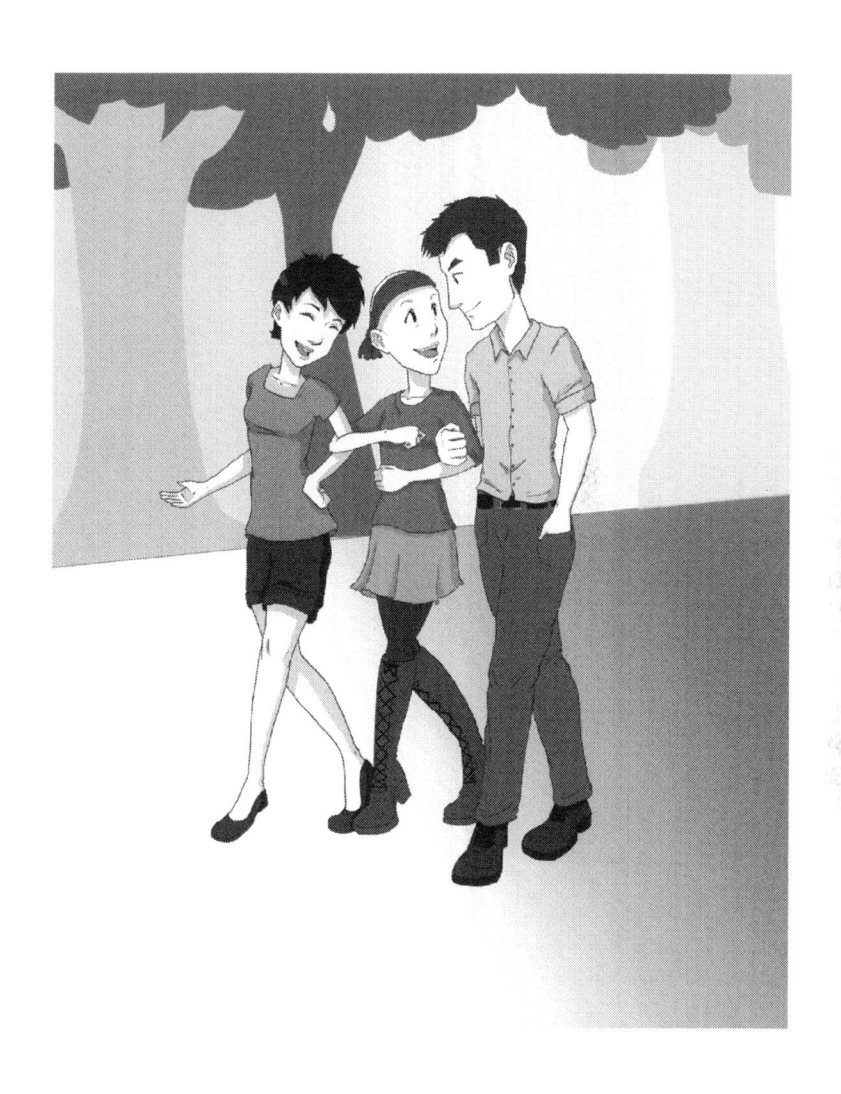

Friends forever. No matter what. We love you!

## LIFE LESSONS

Through my cancer journey I have learned these things.

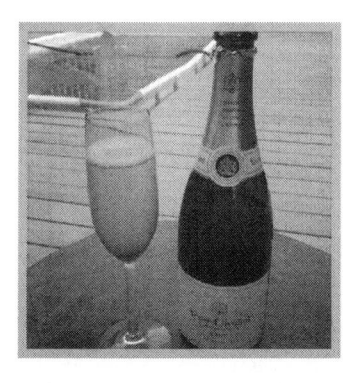

The biggest thing I regret in life is not following my dream. I wanted to be an actor, and I know I would have been a good one, however I was told I should not do that and that I had better skills to develop.

The person who told me that was correct. I have had a very successful business career, always top tier, always an asset and a top performer.

That being said, to this day I long for a career onstage. So as someone who is now looking back on her life I would like to make the following suggestions. Purely my small slice of the pie advice but I think it is pretty accurate.

1). You only live once.

2). Most people do not know how short and fragile their lives could be.

3). When faced with death (or a prescribed death schedule) you only have two choices. To accept it or to fight it. I choose to fight it.

4). I will do everything I want to do no matter how crazy as long as it doesn't hurt another person.

5). I no longer question my weight (which has always been a healthy 120-125lbs) or my wine intake (which is often more than the norm). I stick to the rule of sanity. If I can still bike 5km every day with my dog and still stand after a bottle of champagne, not only am I good, I am happy.

6). I will tell my kids I love them every time I can (I already did this for years). Because for all I know, it could be the last time.

7). Having a faithful loving husband who I adore is worth a million George Clooney's

8). True friends may take a lifetime to find but when you know them, they know you and it is magic.

9). I will never give up living and having fun.

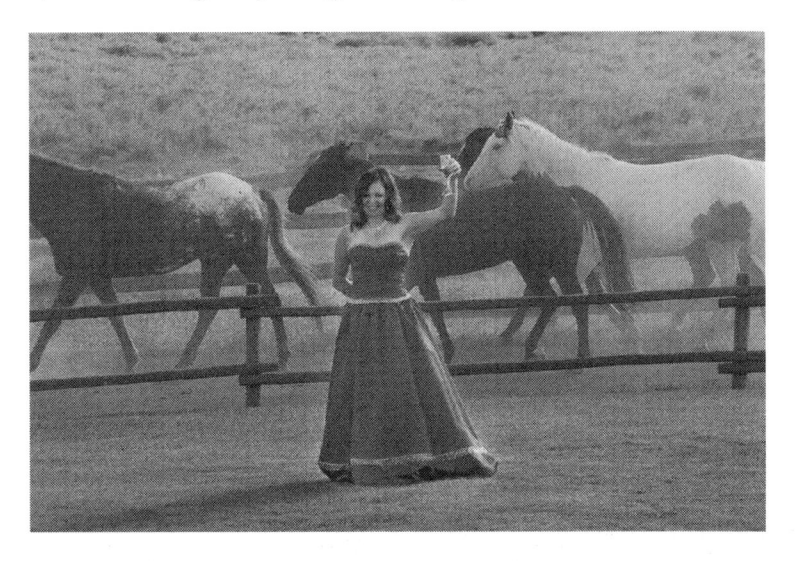

10). I am glad I was someone who always (since I was a child and much to my parents chagrin) lived her life to its fullest. That way I have few regrets.

11). I was born to really rock life and it will take a coffin to stop that natural instinct of mine.

12). Life will go on without me although I warn you all, it won't be as much fun.

13). Get an education so that your choices are not limited when you are older. You never know what amazing imaginative career path you may choose to create.

14). Things are irrelevant. It is the people you love that matter.

15). Life is too short to be with someone who doesn't adore you.

16). Don't underestimate your parents. They will become your greatest loves and your greatest mentors.

17). Giving to others is more joyful than taking.

18). I may not live long, but I have loved and I have loved deeply. I am so grateful for the opportunity to take a risk and pour my heart and soul into loving another person regardless of the outcome. Love is exceptional and will stay with you forever.

19). Tell your parents you love them as often as you can. My mother died too soon and although I believe she knew I loved her, I have since felt a great guilt that I didn't show it enough. My father is my hero and I could never imagine a life without him, yet I still feel I do not express my love and appreciation of him enough. I guess that is a work in progress.

20). Tell your siblings you love them. My brother was ripped from my life far too early. I know deep inside he knew I loved him, that is not the issue. The challenge for me is that I never expressed to my sister how much I loved and respected her. So now due to my negligence we are not as close as I would like. So..... don't wait for trauma to bring you together. Just do it!

21). I did not cause my cancer, it just happened. Which showed me it can happen to anyone. Don't waste your life. Don't save that candle for a special day. Embrace this incredible gift called life. It is wonderful, it has its ups and downs and it may throw you to the curb, but it is far better than the alternative. Death.

22). I would want to trade lives with anyone who is cancer free, but then that person would have my cancer and I am not okay with that. So considering that is not an option, I choose to live out the rest of my life in the following ways:

* I want to have my kids know, respect and love me before I die.
* I want to spend my last few years of life with my husband travelling and living in tropical places (remember I grew up in South Africa).
* I want to leave a legacy of bravery, spirit and fighting so that other people with Inflammatory Breast Cancer or any kind if cancer will fight as hard as I have. One day there will be a cure.
* I want to help people newly diagnosed with cancer in the only way I can which is the Warrior Bag program of love.
* I want to enjoy every day from this one forth in bliss, honesty and integrity.

(And yes to y'all that includes lots of wine for me).

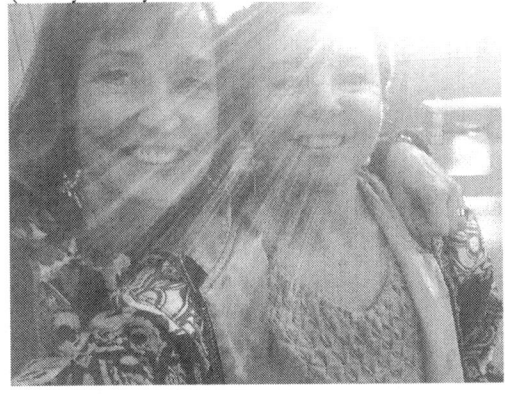

Me enjoying wine with my dear friend Michele

# BEYOND CANCER

Hopefully there will come a day when your cancer will be in remission, or your oncologist will tell you that you show no evidence of disease (NED). This is the day we all dream of and it is a wonderful day, but as you probably know by now. Life will never be the same.

For the first few months you may suffer from depression. This is quite common for cancer patients, especially those who have had a difficult diagnosis and have been through lots of different treatment modalities. Some cousellors have said coming out of cancer is akin to having PTSD, and in a way that is accurate. Your body and your mind have both been though hell and back and it will take a while for you to find your "New Normal".

You will no longer be going from chemo appointment to scan to blood work to radiology etc. There will not be the kind of support you had during your illness. You will be considered "well" and may look well on the outside, but don't worry if you don't feel ready to face the world yet. Your heart still has to heal. The young innocent child that you once were is now gone. You have been touched by cancer and will never be the same. Be kind to yourself and take whatever time you need to return to the world. Don't over do it and make sure you go back slowly so as not to stress your body.

For the first few months after the clean bill of health you will be anxious and worried that the cancer will return. This is completely normal, and as each scan approaches you will get more and more nervous. However, with time, and with each continuous "clear" check up, your worries will begin to cease and you will one day find yourself having gone through an entire day without even thinking about cancer. Imagine that, an entire day where you go about your life simply being and enjoying and not even remembering that you once not so long ago were very sick and did not know what type of future you would have.

Once you reach this point I hope that you have long since

passed this book onto someone else who needs it. I hope that your life is joyous and full and that you never have to face the beast again.

Onwards and Upwards!

To Surviving with Grace!

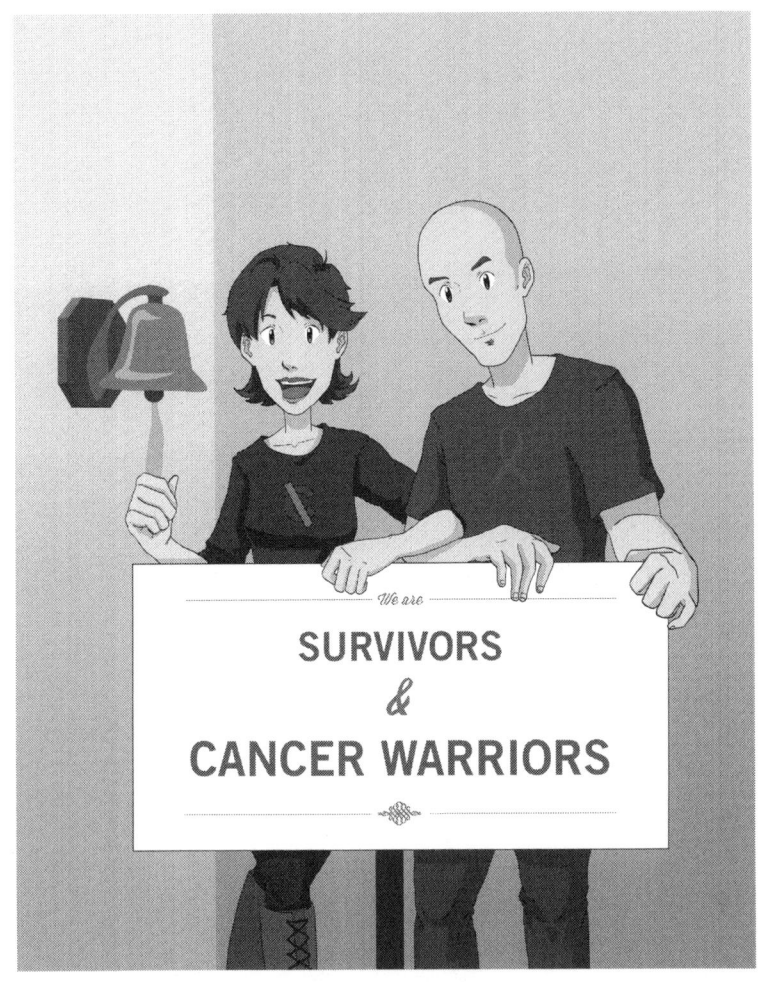

Gabby and Zach

# THE CANCER WARRIOR HANDBOOK

# RESOURCES

The following list of resources is only a short listing of the many places you can go to for information and support during your cancer journey. As future editions of this book comes out, we will be updating this resource section, so please if you find an amazing resource, be it local or online, please contact us on Facebook so we may add it to the next book.

Facebook Resources:

Cancer Warriors Rock!
https://www.facebook.com/groups/472092746218826/

*Ovarian Cancer Together!
https://www.facebook.com/groups/ovariancancertogethergroup/

*Inflammatory Breast Cancer (IBC) Support
https://www.facebook.com/groups/155583871626/

Colon Cancer Alliance
https://www.facebook.com/groups/29075372469/

Lung Cancer Connection
https://www.facebook.com/groups/100537029786/

Prostate and Prostate Cancer Awareness
https://www.facebook.com/groups/44782433175/

*Brain Cancer Family
https://www.facebook.com/groups/111630445593565/

Testicular Cancer Support Group
https://www.facebook.com/groups/4657378483/

Stupid Dumb Breast Cancer
https://www.facebook.com/stupiddumbbreastcancer/

Fuck Cancer
https://www.facebook.com/letsfcancer

Support the Fight Against Breast Cancer
https://www.facebook.com/supportthefight

Team Shan Breast Cancer Awareness for Young Women
https://www.facebook.com/team.shan.ca

Bowel & Cancer Research
https://www.facebook.com/BandC.Research

Kris Carr
https://www.facebook.com/KrisCarr.FanPage

*Indicates a closed group. You will need to request permission to join these groups.

Blogs:

Crazy Sexy Wellness: www.kriscarr.com
Giving Cancer the Boot: www.pammenteryoung.com
Stupid Dumb Breast Cancer: www.supiddumbbreastcancer.com
Suleika's Blog: http://well.blogs.nytimes.com/author/suleika-jaouad/
Nancy's Point: www.nancyspoint.com
Anne Maria Ciccarella: www.chemo-brain.blogspot.ca

## Community Supports:

In some communities they have a local Community Support Services agency that have programs such as community kitchens, visiting volunteers, financial hardship assistance, food banks, free or sliding scale counseling or other health care services. You can try searching the Internet or telephone blue pages.

**Agencies and Wellness Organizations:**

Inspire Health: www.inspirehealth.ca (BC, Canada)
Callanish Society: www.callanish.org
BC Cancer Agency: www.bccanceragency.ca
National Cancer Institute: www.nci.gov
MD Anderson: www.mdanderson.org
Livestrong: www.livestrong.org
Mayo Clinic: www.mayoclinic.com
American Cancer Society: www.cancer.org
Canadian Cancer Society: www.cancer.ca
Best Doctors: www.bestdoctors.com
Best Doctors Canada: www.bestdoctorscanada.com
Unbridling Your Brilliance: www.unbridlingyourbrilliance.com

**Palliative Care**

Palliative means that they don't consider your condition curable - however it may be manageable. In the past a "palliative" treatment program seemed to imply you were going to pass away shortly. However many treatments for metastatic cancer are now given with the expectation you will manage with cancer as a chronic disease for longer periods of time. Your team can provide treatments to manage symptoms and improve quality of life.

Palliative Care - End of Life Support

Most provinces offer supports in home and in hospice for end of life care. Contact your local health unit for information.

British Columbia Palliative Care benefits

In BC your doctor fills out the Palliative Care Benefits package when your treatments are no longer successful and they estimate you have lest than 6 months to live. Please know that they must have your informed consent to do so and it does not have to be a "death sentence" once signed. You have a right to change your mind, seek alternative treatments and never, ever give up HOPE if that's what you want.

The benefits are that many home care supplies and medications are fully covered if they are on the provincial formulary. You will be connected with a Palliative Care case manager who can work with your doctors to ensure your symptoms are being controlled. You can gain access to major equipment such as lifts and hospital beds and hospice facilities. Home care nurses, OT's and PT's, hospice volunteers and home support providers can visit and assist you in your own home.

http://www.health.gov.bc.ca/pharmacare/outgoing/palliative.html

# WAGE REPLACEMENT

Insert Wage replacement - information for Canada only

**Employee benefits**:
Ask your employer (human resources/employee engagement)
- ☐ Sick time
- ☐ Short term illness/disability
- ☐ Long term disability
- ☐ You may also be eligible for payout of prior vacation days accumulated depending on your employer

## **Provincial**

**Ministry of Social Development and Social Innovation BC**

(This Ministry name changes often and varies between provinces)

You can apply for income assistance or disability assistance as a "last resort." They have programs to assist with childcare, and return to work if you are eligible and receiving their benefits.

http://www.hsd.gov.bc.ca/bcea.htm

## **Federal**

**Employment Insurance**

Temporary financial assistance while you are undergoing treatment or waiting for long-term benefits to be approved.

http://www.servicecanada.gc.ca/eng/ei/application/employmentinsurance.shtml

**CPP disability**

If you are going to be off work for a long time or have a serious condition it may be worth applying for CPP. Some LTD plans will insist you apply and will deduct any money paid from their share. However, there are advantages to CPP disability including financial and vocational support on a return to work and childcare benefits.

http://www.servicecanada.gc.ca/eng/isp/cpp/disaben.shtml

## **Vocational Rehabilitation**

Returning to work after cancer can be challenging. If you are returning to your previous job, you may be able to return on a light or gradual schedule over several weeks. Perhaps you are looking for a new job or career so you can better manage with the residual effects of cancer.

If you have been away from work for a long time or have a physically demanding job it may be best to do a fitness or work conditioning program designed to help build up your tolerances for work. Sometimes your employer or LTD provider will pay for "Occupational Rehab" or a personal trainer with experience in return to work.

And don't forget the cognitive and emotional aspects of cancer. A vocational counsellor or Occupational Therapist (See yellow pages) can help coordinate your return to work successfully using strategies.

Some Cancer treatment centers have vocational counselling.

http://www.bccancer.bc.ca/PPI/copingwithcancer/emotional/Work+Related+Issues.htm

A note to the reader:

This book is a work in progress. I would love your help adding to the ABC's section and if you wish to contribute a story for future editions, please contact me on my blog or Facebook page:

Facebook: www.facebook.com/MichellePammenterYoung
Blog: www.pammenteryoung.com

# EXCERPT FROM "THE YEAR I DIED"

## PROLOGUE

I flip my legs over the side of the bed and rush the twelve or so feet to the ensuite bathroom, throw myself on my knees and just manage to grab the toilet bowl before the surge starts. Over and over again I retch, at first there is a little bit to come up. I haven't been eating much lately, so I'm surprised there is anything. Then for the next ten minutes I yoyo between lying on the floor exhausted, to hanging onto the toilet retching, my body wracked by dry heaves.

Finally the nausea subsides and I quietly curl up into a ball on the carpeted bathroom floor breathing shallowly. "I can't take this anymore," I think as the slow sound of a deep howl begins to escape my throat. The feeling of nausea is replaced with something far worse: a deep sense of pain, of loss, of regret and of horror. How can this be happening to me? Surely this is some horrific nightmare from which I will soon awaken and give a sigh of relief that it's over. I hold onto my knees and sob and sob, feeling my chest heave and the palms of my hands ache. I'm not sure why, but my palms always ache when I'm experiencing heartbreak, although this is not heartbreak, this is something beyond heartbreak.

I cry out of sadness, out of frustration, how, how can this be happening to me? I have a great life. It's always been good. I mean, I've had my ups and downs, but really when I look around me at what I've been able to achieve and how I live, I consider myself pretty lucky. Perhaps, some would say I've worked for it, and yes perhaps I have, I am a driver after all - Miss Type A personality - always wanting to be at the top. Is that why this is happening to me? Was life too good? Did I do something to make this happen to me? I lie here on the floor questioning myself, questioning my life, breaking it down into chapters and moments to try and find the fatal flaw. The thing I did to make it all go so wrong, or perhaps the things I have done that contributed to this.

I think back to my early childhood, I was born in South Africa in the sixties when it was still relatively safe there. I had a great childhood. I was adopted at a very young age and my parents always loved me. They may have been incredibly strict and sometimes over the top with their rules, but they raised me well and showed me the value of working hard as well as enjoying life. When I was quite young we lived in Kloof in what was then the Natal Province of South Africa. It was an incredible place to live; I will always remember the warm winds that used to circle our house. My father had built a beautiful house for us; it was round, like a doughnut. We loved that house my brother, sister and I. Yes, I had a brother, who was adopted when I was one and a sister, also adopted when I was almost four. We did have another baby brother, Bussy was his name, he was only a foster child and unfortunately his family took him back after four years. That was the first time I recall my mother having her heart broken. I don't think she ever recovered from that and in some ways that event tore the family apart, ever so slightly. Not enough that you would notice, but enough that there was a tiny fissure which would eventually grow over the years until it cracked, but that is another story.

My brother Sean and my sister Marie and I were typical kids; we loved playing outside, loved getting into trouble, and of course fought like all normal siblings do. We were very lucky in that we travelled to Germany a lot as children to spend Christmas with our cousins, as well as fortunate enough to spend many trips with our family in and around South Africa. Our education was both worldly and practical. My mother Jackie stayed home with us and although she was a typical mother of the sixties when children should be seen and not heard, she also spent some wonderful times with us. I recall sitting on her lap in the evening as she read us our bedtime stories. After the story I'd ask, "Mummy, tell me the story about how you adopted me", and she'd smile and hug me tighter and tell me the lovely story. The story about how she wanted children so very badly, but couldn't have any of her own, and then she got a call that there was a little baby girl in Durban and would she like to come and meet her. Mummy said that the minute she laid eyes on me she loved me and wanted me and so I always felt chosen and blessed.

So why, if I was chosen and blessed and loved did I end up here, curled up in a ball on my bathroom floor begging for a different life. Oh well I think, as I pick myself back up. I must go on. I cannot quit. I must continue to work through this, if not for myself, then for my children and my husband and my family, my dear mother and father and my younger brother and sister who love me.

I check the time on my iPhone before I climb back into bed. It is three in the morning, Vancouver time, and another sleepless night I think, as I lie down exhausted from sickness and the emotional breakdown I have just had. At least it is officially the shortest night of the year. I close my eyes and feel myself gently drifting off into sleep; I relish this, a place where for a short time I can forget. My last thought before I slip into dreamland is "I guess it can't get any worse than this". Boy was I wrong.

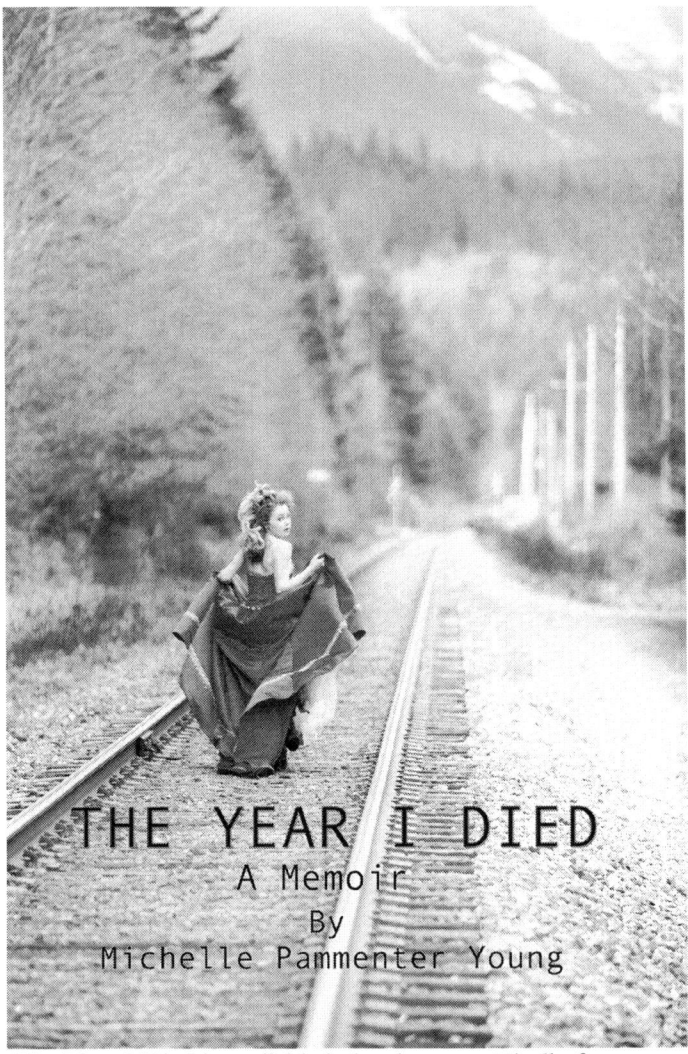

# THE YEAR I DIED
### A Memoir
### By
### Michelle Pammenter Young

The Year I Died is available in hardcopy or Kindle format at:
www.amazon.com/Year-Died-Michelle-Pammenter-Young/dp/1482714930
Photography © Gadbois Photograpy
www.gadboisphotography.ca

# ABOUT THE AUTHOR

Michelle Pammenter Young is a financial advisor turned writer and cancer warrior. In June 2012 Michelle was diagnosed with Inflammatory Breast Cancer, a rare and very serious form of breast cancer. Michelle started a blog to document her journey, which eventually became her first book "The Year I Died" an actual account of her harrowing journey through cancer, death and family tragedy. After the success of her first book, and looking to help others going through the cancer journey, Michelle began work on "The Cancer Warrior Handbook". She is also actively involved in "The Warrior Bag Program" a way to give back to cancer patients in her community. Michelle grew up in South Africa and now lives in British Columbia, Canada with her husband, two children, a cat and a dog named Waldo.